18/03/19
05/04/19
29/04/19

Cambridgeshire Libraries, Archives and Information Service

This book is due for return on or before the latest date shown above, but may be renewed up to three times unless it has been requested by another customer.

Books can be renewed –
In person at your local library

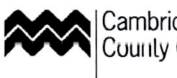 Cambridgeshire County Council

Online www.cambridgeshire.gov.uk/library

Please note that charges are made on overdue books.

10010010496678

UNDERSTANDING AND DEALING WITH HEART DISEASE

Copyright © Keith Souter, 2014

Illustrations © Keith Souter

All rights reserved.

No part of this book may be reproduced by any means, nor transmitted, nor translated into a machine language, without the written permission of the publishers.

Keith Souter has asserted his right to be identified as the author of this work in accordance with sections 77 and 78 of the Copyright, Designs and Patents Act 1988.

Condition of Sale
This book is sold subject to the condition that it shall not, by way of trade or otherwise, be lent, resold, hired out or otherwise circulated in any form of binding or cover other than that in which it is published and without a similar condition including this condition being imposed on the subsequent purchaser.

Vie Books is an imprint of Summersdale

Summersdale Publishers Ltd
46 West Street
Chichester
West Sussex
PO19 1RP
UK

www.summersdale.com

Printed and bound by CPI Group (UK) Ltd

ISBN: 978-1-84953-557-1

Cambridgeshire Libraries	
10010010496678	
Askews & Holts	27-Nov-2017
616.12	£8.99

Substantial discounts on bulk quantities of Summersdale books are available to corporations, professional associations and other organisations. For details contact general enquiries: telephone: +44 (0) 1243 771107, fax: +44 (0) 1243 786300 or email: enquiries@summersdale.com.

Disclaimer
Every effort has been made to ensure that the information in this book is accurate and current at the time of publication. The author and the publisher cannot accept responsibility for any misuse or misunderstanding of any information contained herein, or any loss, damage or injury, be it health, financial or otherwise, suffered by any individual or group acting upon or relying on information contained herein. None of the opinions or suggestions in this book are intended to replace medical opinion. If you have concerns about your health, please seek professional advice.

For my brother-in-law, Phil

Acknowledgements

I would like to thank Isabel Atherton, my wonderful agent at Creative Authors, for helping to bring this book to fruition. Thanks also to Claire Plimmer at Summersdale who commissioned the title and read the first draft, and to my editor, Abbie Headon for the helpful suggestions and deft work with the editorial pen. Thanks also to Ray Hamilton, my copy-editor, who helped to smooth out the manuscript. It has been a great pleasure to work with them all.

Finally, a huge thank you to Dr Richard Sloan, a fellow GP who is also a physiologist, for taking the time to write the foreword. I particularly valued his opinion since he was able to consider the book from his perspective as a GP and as a scientist.

Keith Souter

Contents

Foreword 9
by Dr Richard Sloan, MBE, MB, BS, BSc, PhD, FRCGP

Introduction 11

PART ONE: UNDERSTANDING HEART DISEASE 15
Your heart deserves respect

Chapter 1: Understand the heart 18

Basic heart and circulation facts
The circulatory system
What the ancients thought about the heart and circulation
The rise of anatomy
The circulatory system described
What happens during the cardiac cycle as the heart beats
The conducting system of the heart
The blood

Chapter 2: The different types of cardiovascular disease 38

Let's get the names right
Cardiovascular disease
Heart disease
Coronary heart disease
Congenital heart disease
Valvular heart disease
Cardiomyopathy
Stroke
Peripheral artery disease
Aortic artery disease

Chapter 3: Hardening of the arteries 50

Arteriosclerosis and atherosclerosis
The anatomical structure of the arteries

The pathological process – what actually happens
Thrombus formation
The consequences of atherosclerosis
Blockage of arteries causes two types of problem
Anatomical consequences

Chapter 4: Hypertension (high blood pressure).....................60

What is hypertension?
The dangers of hypertension
What is blood pressure?
The discovery of blood pressure
The causes of hypertension
The way the body controls blood pressure

Chapter 5: How coronary heart disease manifests itself.....................78

The different presentations
Chest pain – the commonest symptom
Angina pectoris
Acute coronary syndrome

Chapter 6: Heart failure.....................88

The many causes of heart failure
The different forms of heart failure

Chapter 7: Congenital heart disease.....................99

The causes of congenital heart disease
Genetic problems
Infections during pregnancy
Diabetes mellitus
Alcohol
Iatrogenic
The symptoms of congenital heart disease
Acyanotic conditions
Cyanotic conditions

Chapter 8: Valvular heart disease.....................109

The four heart valves
The causes of valvular heart disease

The symptoms of valvular heart disease
Mitral valve disease
Aortic valve disease
Endocarditis – the problem that valvular heart disease can cause
Assessment
Treatment of valvular heart disease
Heart surgery

Chapter 9: Other diseases of the heart..118

Cardiomyopathy
Types of cardiomyopathy
Myocarditis
Pericarditis

PART TWO: DEALING WITH HEART DISEASE......................................124

You can look after your heart

Chapter 10: Understanding your risk of having a heart attack........126

Risk factors for coronary heart disease
Non-modifiable risk factors
Modifiable risk factors
Cardiovascular risk assessment

Chapter 11: What could this chest pain be? Is it angina?..................142

The symptoms to look out for
Angina – a general description
Your GP
The ECG
It isn't necessarily angina – the differential diagnosis
Further investigations to be carried out
Treatment of angina

Chapter 12: Heart attacks – what happens...162

Emergency care
In hospital
Drugs on discharge from hospital

Chapter 13: Managing heart failure.........................176

The range of symptoms
Physical signs the doctor will look for
Pinpointing the problem
Treatment of heart failure
Devices
Surgical treatment
Heart transplantation

Chapter 14: Irregular hearts.........................192

Symptoms of arrhythmias
Causes of arrhythmias
Diagnosis
Types of arrhythmias
Drugs used to treat arrhythmias
Devices

Chapter 15: After a heart attack.........................210

Cardiac rehabilitation
Work
Driving
Sex life
Emotional recovery
The life cycle

Chapter 16: Managing hypertension.........................217

Diagnosis of blood pressure
Special considerations
Investigations
Management of blood pressure

Chapter 17: The life cycle.........................225

The life cycle – a summary
Use the life cycle to sketch out your life
The sphere of emotion
The sphere of the mind
The sphere of behaviour

The sphere of lifestyle
  The sphere of body
  Putting it all together

Chapter 18: A healthy diet and taking some exercise..........................241

  Diet
  The Mediterranean diet
  A short lesson about fats and oils
  Avoid junk food
  Obesity
  Salt intake
  Antioxidants
  Five fruit and veg a day – eat the rainbow way
  Take some exercise
  Types of exercise

Finally, it is not all doom and gloom!..254

Appendix: Cardiopulmonary resuscitation (CPR)..............................255
Glossary..257
Directory of useful addresses..264
References...270

Foreword

By Dr Richard Sloan, MBE, MB, BS, BSc, PhD, FRCGP

Keith Souter and I worked as general practitioners for many years in the Wakefield district of West Yorkshire, England. Each of us has witnessed the amazing and fantastic advances in the diagnosis and treatment of the many and varied diseases that can affect the heart. In the early 1970s, when I started working as a GP, it was acceptable for a heart attack to be dealt with in the patient's home. A consultant could be asked to visit and undertake an ECG, and that was probably the only investigation carried out apart from measuring the blood pressure and pulse. In 2014, if you have chest pain which sounds as though it could be a heart attack, the initial assessment will probably be made by paramedics arriving in an emergency ambulance. You would then be rushed, preferably, to a heart attack centre and a firm diagnosis would be made, followed by thrombolysis (clot busting) and then possible angioplasty (the insertion of a stent) to keep the blocked artery open.

This book is the third in a series called *Understanding and Dealing with…* The subjects for the first two were stroke and depression.

Part 1 of the book is a thoroughly researched description of the anatomy and physiology of the heart, followed by the pathology of the many diseases that can affect the heart and circulation. The description of how ancient civilisations viewed the heart and pulse, along with the work of William Harvey, makes one realise how the science of heart disease has advanced over the centuries, and that further advances will be made in the future. The clear explanation of the terminology that is commonly used by the medical profession should be invaluable to patients wanting to understand their particular heart disease better.

Part 2 gives advice on how to prevent certain heart diseases by means of diet, exercise, etc. The management and treatment of the diseases affecting the heart and circulation is described in a way that will be most helpful to anyone being investigated or suffering from one of these. The advantages of the Mediterranean diet and the deficiencies of the British diet are examined. There is a detailed explanation of the roles of different fats, and there is also an explanation as to how to calculate the risk of having a heart attack.

In my opinion, one of the most important sections of this book is how to deal with recovering after a heart attack. This includes emotional recovery and there is a whole chapter on 'the life cycle', a tool Dr Souter has developed and used successfully with patients when he worked as a general practitioner. It helps patients to look at their lives and develop self-help strategies. The chapter showing us how to use this tool also completes the books on depression and stroke.

Not only is this book a must for patients with heart disease but also I feel there should be a copy in every medical library as it is an excellent reference book for healthcare professionals and students.

Introduction

The heart is one of the most important organs in the body. It supplies every organ and tissue of the body with oxygen and nutrients, which are needed to maintain life.

Cardiovascular disease, often abbreviated to CVD, is the name given to include all the diseases of the heart and the circulation. Within it there are several types of heart disease, including coronary heart disease, congenital heart disease, valvular heart disease and cardiomyopathy. We shall touch on all of them in this book, but the main emphasis throughout is going to be on coronary heart disease and its various manifestations. This is by far the largest and the commonest group.

Coronary heart disease, often abbreviated to CHD, is the largest cause of death in the UK today. It causes the deaths of about 82,000 people each year. One man in five dies from it, compared with one woman in eight. Those are stark enough figures, but there is growing concern that, after several years in which we have seen a decline in the number of people suffering with coronary heart disease, and in the death rates from it, we may begin to see a rise in the future. The problem is that obesity rates are rising, and with obesity comes the increased risk of developing problems like hypertension and coronary heart disease.

There are various ways that coronary heart disease can manifest itself. It can cause angina, or chest pain on exertion. It can cause heart failure. It can produce palpitations and abnormal heart rhythms. And, most importantly, it can cause heart attacks. A severe heart attack can result in the heart stopping, which is known as a cardiac arrest. Unless the heart is restarted very soon, death will result.

But it is not all bad news. Modern medicine has much to offer people who have coronary heart disease.

The aim of this book is to provide basic information to help readers understand coronary heart disease and the way that it can affect the heart. If you understand the nature of the condition then you can work with your doctor to deal with the symptoms or whatever condition results from it. This can be of value not only to the person with the problem, but to members of the family who may find that they have to be involved in the care of that person. It also gives information about how to spot risk factors that the reader or other members of their family should be aware of, in order to prevent themselves from developing angina, or heart failure, or having a heart attack.

The book naturally falls into two parts. The first part is all about understanding the conditions, so the first few chapters will describe the heart and how it works as a pump in order to supply the rest of the body with precious blood containing oxygen and nutrients. This will be followed by chapters outlining the pathological process of arteriosclerosis and hypertension, and how they may cause the various problems that can result.

Wherever appropriate, statistics and key points will be featured in order to put problems into context. For example, Chapter 2 will describe the different types of cardiovascular disease and Chapter 3 will outline the various problems that can be caused by arteriosclerosis (hardening of the arteries).

The second part of the book is about dealing with the aftermath of having a heart attack or how to deal with angina or heart failure. And it will also be looking at ways to avoid problems developing, e.g. through the management of blood pressure.

We will cover all of the investigations that need to be carried out when coronary heart disease is either suspected or confirmed. We will also focus on risk factors for various problems, including the risk of coronary heart disease in other members of the family, and what one can do to reduce those risks. And, most importantly, we shall be looking at the symptoms and signs that occur in angina, heart attacks and other manifestations of heart disease.

It is appreciated that there are many medical terms that may be new to you, so a glossary explaining the main terms is present at the back of the book.

Some basic facts

- In 2011, there were estimated to be 1.1 million men in the UK with angina.
- 6.5 per cent of men in the UK have heart disease.
- 4 per cent of women in the UK have heart disease.
- The rate rises with age. One in three men and one in four women over the age of 75 will have heart disease.
- Men are two to three times more at risk than women *until* the menopause. The female hormones seem to have a protective effect and after the menopause that protective role is lost, so the rates are then far closer.
- Heart and circulatory diseases are the UK's biggest killers. In 2007, cardiovascular disease caused 34 per cent of deaths in the UK (193,000 people).
- According to the continuously updated Scottish Morbidity Study,

there are a total of 96,000 new cases of angina per year in Scotland alone.

- At the time of writing, the cost of healthcare in the UK as the result of cardiovascular disease is £1.7 billion per year.

PART ONE

UNDERSTANDING HEART DISEASE

Your heart deserves respect

The human heart has been the subject of study for poets, philosophers and theologians for millennia. It has been regarded at times as the seat of the soul, or the organ of thought, or the place where we feel our emotions. Doctors have also been concerned about it for the same length of time, for it has been known since antiquity that its function is necessary for life to continue. It has also been known that malfunction produces a range of symptoms including palpitations and angina attacks, or collapse through a sudden 'heart attack'.

The heart is a muscular pump that is the size of a clenched fist in childhood and the size of two fists in adulthood. It never stops working. Throughout your life it beats, pumping blood to all parts of the body. It pumps blood to the lungs where it picks up oxygen and is returned to the heart, which then pumps oxygen-rich blood to the rest of the body.

Over the years we have been able to delineate many factors that are bad for your heart health and which cause coronary heart disease.

That is, we have been able to determine what foods are more likely to boost blood-cholesterol levels and promote the laying down of fat deposits in the coronary arteries, the blood vessels which supply the heart itself with oxygen. And, of course, smoking has been associated with an increased risk of dying from heart attacks ever since Doll and Hill published their landmark papers on lung cancer and smoking in a sample population of British doctors in the 1950s. [1] [2] [3]

Medical science has made great strides and your doctor can now perform a range of checks, which can give you a measure of your risk of having a heart attack from coronary heart disease. The fact is that it is generally possible to reduce your risk. That means that you can reduce your risk of dying from this condition. All that it demands is that you respect your heart and adopt a lifestyle that is geared towards the maintenance of a long and healthy life.

Chapter 1

Understand the heart

The heart is the main organ of the circulatory system. It pumps blood to every part of the body and it does so every minute of your life. If the heart stops beating, your brain is deprived of oxygen. Your brain can only manage about six minutes before its cells start to die. Indeed, unless your heart is restarted and an adequate pulse is established, your death will occur within that same timescale.

If a coronary artery, one of the main blood vessels that supply the heart itself with blood, is blocked, then the heart muscle supplied by it will die in around 5–10 minutes. This is referred to as a myocardial infarction.

Nowadays we are aware of the heart's prime role as a pump, yet for millennia the understanding of its purpose was quite sketchy. Since people experience a quickening of the heart when they are excited or afraid, or even a sinking feeling in the chest when they are alarmed, it is not surprising that in antiquity the heart came to be thought of as an organ related to the emotions and the soul.

It is worth following the theories that have been held about the heart and the blood vessels over the centuries, in order to show just how our knowledge about this majestic organ developed, but first let us look at the basic facts as we now know them.

Basic heart and circulation facts

- The heart is a double-action pump.
- It has four chambers: two upper atria and two lower ventricles.
- The right ventricle pumps blood to the lungs to collect oxygen and bring it back to the heart.
- The left ventricle pumps oxygenated blood to the rest of the body.
- The average adult female heart weighs about 8 ounces.
- The average adult male heart weighs about 10–12 ounces.
- The adult heart is about the size of two fists placed side by side.
- The heart beats on average 70 times a minute, that is 100,000 times a day, 35 million times a year and on average 2.5 billion times in a lifetime.
- There are 8 pints of blood in the circulation.
- Arteries carry blood away from the heart.
- Veins carry blood back to the heart.
- If you put all of your blood vessels together to make a long single tube, it would stretch 60,000 miles, which would take you more than twice around the world.
- The heart is a pumping muscle of incredible strength, which could:
    - lift a medium-sized car
    - squirt a jet of blood 30 feet
    - pump a million barrels of blood in a lifetime.

The circulatory system

The circulatory system consists of the heart and the blood vessels that carry blood around the body to all of its organs and tissues. The heart is the main organ of the circulatory system. It is located in the thorax, slightly on the left side of the midline of the body. As a result the left lung is slightly smaller than the right in order to accommodate it.

Effectively, the heart is like two pumps joined together; the left side of the heart receives oxygenated (oxygen-rich) blood from the lungs and pumps it out to the organs and tissues. This is called the systemic circulation.

The brain, the liver, the kidneys and all of the major organs (including the lungs, which supply oxygen to the blood pumped to it from the right side of the heart) receive their supply of blood from the systemic circulation.

The right side of the heart receives deoxygenated (oxygen-depleted) blood from the tissues and pumps it out to the lungs to collect more oxygen. This is called the pulmonary circulation.

KEY POINTS

- The heart muscle has to have its own blood supply, since it cannot extract oxygen from the blood that flows through it.
- The lungs have to have their own supply of systemic oxygen-rich blood, since they also have to have oxygen and nutrients.

Arteries carry oxygenated blood to the organs and tissues to nourish them. Veins carry deoxygenated blood back to the heart, in order to be pumped to the lungs to receive more oxygen.

Arterioles are the very smallest arteries. They link up in the tissues with capillaries.

Capillaries are tiny thread-like blood vessels that join the arterial circulation to the venous circulation, and which feed the tissues.

That, in a nutshell, is a description of the circulation. But we shall now have a look at how we came to understand all these facts (and then we shall return to develop a clearer picture of the heart and circulation).

What the ancients thought about the heart and circulation

In Ancient Babylon physicians believed that there were two types of blood vessel, which carried two types of blood. This idea must have come from empirical observation of the colour of blood, for they thought that arterial blood was the blood of the day, and that venous blood was the blood of the night. And indeed, arterial blood is bright and venous blood is darker.

The Ancient Egyptians, of course, left us a great deal of information about their lives, not only in artefacts of daily life in their tombs, but also in actual written records. We know that they considered the soul to be made up of five separate components, each of which resided in a different part of the person. The *ib* was the heart and was believed to be the centre of their emotions, thoughts, will and consciousness. It was considered to be the most important of organs, far more so than the brain, which was pulled out through the nose and discarded during the embalming process of mummification.

It was their belief that the heart was formed in the developing baby from a single drop of the mother's blood. Also, after death, they believed that in order for the soul to pass through the underworld to enjoy the afterlife, it had to pass the 'weighing of the heart' ceremony. This was presided over by Osiris, the god of the underworld. The heart was weighed by the jackal-headed god Anubis, against the feather of Maat, or truth. If the heart was too heavy, as the result of sins and bad deeds, it would be cast aside to be devoured by the monster Ammit, who had the head of a crocodile, the torso of a lion and the hindquarters of a hippopotamus.

There are several medical and surgical papyri, which give us information about the extent of the Egyptians' knowledge of the function of the heart and about conditions affecting the heart. The three principal ones are all named after their discoverers.

The Edwin Smith papyrus

This has been dated back to 1600 BC, but is thought to have been based on a copy from the Old Kingdom of Egypt in around 3000 BC. It is attributed to the priest-physician Imhotep, who was also the grand vizier to King Djoser. Apart from being a physician, he was an engineer and an architect and is thought to have built the famous step-pyramid at Saqqara. In the papyrus the heart is described as being at the centre of a network of vessels, called *metu*. Fascinatingly, the pulse is also described and associated with the heart.

The Ebers papyrus

This has been dated to 1550 BC. It also describes the heart and its position in the left side of the chest. It also mentions the vessels, or *metu*, but describes many more than in the Edwin Smith papyrus.

The Brugsch papyrus

This is also known as the Greater Berlin papyrus. It is dated to around 1300 BC. Much of it is similar to the Ebers papyrus, but it goes on to describe the veins.

The Greeks later took medicine to a higher level. Hippocrates (*c*.460–*c*.370 BC) was an Ancient Greek physician, commonly regarded as the 'father of medicine'. He was the first physician to reject superstition and demonic possession as causes for illness, instead proposing that illness was due to an imbalance of four humors, or vital fluids. These were blood, phlegm, black bile and yellow bile. This was to remain the dominant medical theory until towards the end of the Renaissance in the seventeenth century.

In his extensive writings, known collectively as the *Corpus Hippocraticum*, he described the Greeks' view of anatomy, disease and treatment. In the book *Peri Kardies*[4], he described the heart thus:

In shape the heart is like a pyramid, in colour dark red, and it is surrounded by a smooth covering, and in this there is a small amount of urine-like fluid, so that you think the heart rests in a bladder.

Here he is describing what the heart actually does look like and the pericardium, which is the sac that envelops it.

In other works[5] he goes on to describe the valves of the heart as well as heart failure, rheumatic fever, cardiac pain, Adams-Stokes syndrome (sudden episodes of faintness sometimes associated with seizures or fits, caused by a slowing of the heart rhythm) and Cheyne-Stokes respiration (abnormal breathing patterns), as well as techniques of abdominal and thoracic paracentesis (the removal of fluid from the body), all of which makes it clear that he recognised that the heart was subject to disease and that it would produce certain symptoms and signs as a result.

THE PULSE OF LIFE

The pulse has been recognised as a fundamental and measurable sign of health or illness by every culture in the world. The earliest references to it are to be found in the Edwin Smith and Ebers papyri, the two texts on medicine and surgery from Ancient Egypt referred to above. There are specific hieroglyphs for measuring the pulse at the wrist, and instructions on how to assess it by using a water clock made from an earthenware vessel with a hole in the bottom through which water escaped drop by drop.

The Chinese also described the importance of taking the pulse as early as 2700 BC. Their concept of it was far subtler, in that it related (and still relates) to their unique concept of how the body works. Essentially, in Chinese medicine each of the organs is associated with a meridian or channel through which energy flows. These 12 meridians can all be assessed by examining the wrist and feeling the pulse with light, medium and firm pressure.

The Ancient Greeks referred to the pulse as *sphygmos*, from which we get our word 'sphygmomanometer' or blood pressure recorder. They described a slow pulse as *bradysphygic* and a fast one as *tachysphygic*.

Although the Egyptians used a water clock and the Romans developed hourglasses to try to measure the pulse, it was not until the Renaissance that a more practical method was developed. Interestingly, this came about through the work of the genius Galileo Galilei, who designed a clock with a pendulum that he called a *pulsogium*. He developed the idea from a principle he discovered in 1583 by timing the oscillations of a chandelier on the altar of the Cathedral of Pisa against his own pulse.

Over the next century pulse clocks of greater sophistication were developed by Santorio Santorio and Christiaan Huygens, but it was not until the eighteenth century that watches capable of measuring minutes and seconds could be adapted to the purpose. In 1707 Sir John Floyer, a Staffordshire physician, invented a small pulse watch and published a landmark book entitled *The Physician's Pulse Watch*. We still use his technique to feel the pulse of life.

The rise of anatomy

Although the Egyptians practised embalming and mummification, it was done as preparation of the body for the afterlife, rather than for medical study.

In the second century the Greek physician Claudius Galenus of Pergamum (c. AD 131–201), better known as Galen, performed several dissections on animals and accurately described many of the organs of the body. He described the function of the nerves, examined the structures of the eyes, ears, larynx and reproductive organs. He taught that 'psychic gases and humours' flowed through the body into the ventricles of the brain, thereby allowing for the development of mental functions.

After that, the Church banned the anatomical dissection of the body and it was not until the sixteenth century that further advances in knowledge about the body were made. Andreas Vesalius (AD 1514–1564) was a Flemish anatomist who demonstrated that Galen and other early anatomists had been incorrect in some of their conclusions. In 1543 he wrote the first anatomically accurate medical textbook, *De Humani Corporis Fabrica* (*On the Fabric of the Human Body*), which was complete with precise illustrations.

Vesalius observed that there was a difference between the blood in arteries and the blood in veins. He thought that the heart manufactured arterial blood and that the liver manufactured venous blood, both types being sent to the extremities of the body by some sort of sucking mechanism of the heart and the liver. When the blood reached its target, it was used up.

It was an explanation, but it was the wrong one.

William Harvey and the circulation of blood

William Harvey (1578–1657) was a physician and anatomist who fought in the English Civil War and who was court physician to three kings of England. After graduating from Cambridge University, he went to study medicine and anatomy at the University of Padua.

He did not think that Vesalius's theory of blood being manufactured by the heart and the liver was logical. Simple arithmetic showed that a huge amount of blood would have to be produced and used up in a short period of time.

After extensive experimentation on animals, he came to the conclusion that there was a constant amount of blood and that it was in continuous circulation, pumped by the heart through the blood vessels.

Harvey announced his discovery of the circulation of the blood in 1616, and in 1628 he published his work *Exercitatio Anatomica de Motu Cordis et Sanguinis in Animalibus* (*An Anatomical Exercise on the Motion of the Heart and Blood in Animals*). It was the most significant piece of medical research ever written and laid the foundation for the scientific study of medicine.

He proposed that blood flowed through the heart in two separate loops, a pulmonary circulation going to the lungs and another, a systemic circulation, going to the organs and extremities.

It was a correct explanation and it gave a good idea of how the circulation worked – yet it was incomplete.

The complete picture

Harvey had worked in Padua under another anatomist known as Fabricius, who had helped him to understand the function of the valves in veins (there are no valves in arteries). As they only worked in one direction, Harvey concluded that they were designed to allow blood to flow towards the heart, but *not* in the other direction. This suggested that blood flowed around and around the body and that the two circulations (arterial and venous) were in some way linked.

Although this gave a good idea of the circulation, Harvey was unable to explain how the two circulations joined up in the tissues. He speculated that there was a means by which they exchanged some vital principle, which happened to be oxygen, but he did not know how.

In 1661, Marcello Malpighi (1628–1694), an Italian doctor, published the results of his experiments on the microscopic examination of the anatomy of a frog's lung. He reported on his findings of *capillaries*, the tiny blood vessels that link the arteries to the veins. This was the missing link that Harvey had been looking for. The complete circulation of the blood had been discovered!

The circulatory system described

History lesson over, we can now describe the nature of the circulatory system. It consists of a double-action pump, which supplies oxygen to all of the tissues of the body via the arteries. It receives blood back from the tissues through our veins and pumps it out again to the lungs to receive more oxygen, which is then pumped again to the tissues.

KEY POINTS ABOUT THE HEART

- The heart is a hollow muscular pump.
- It has four chambers. The two upper ones are called the atria, which pass blood into the two lower chambers, called the ventricles.
- The singular term used when describing just one of the heart's upper chambers is 'atrium', from the Latin meaning 'welcoming hall'. 'Ventricle' also originates from a Latin word meaning 'little belly' or 'stomach'.

- Effectively, the heart is like two pumps joined together; the left side of the heart receives oxygenated (oxygen-rich) blood from the lungs and pumps it out to the tissues. This is called the 'systemic circulation'.
- The right side receives deoxygenated (oxygen-depleted) blood from the tissues and pumps it out to the lungs to collect more oxygen. This is called the 'pulmonary circulation'.
- There are four valves in the heart, whose purpose is to ensure that blood flows through the heart in the right direction between the four chambers.

The valves within the heart are of two types:

- Two atrioventricular (AV) valves which allow blood to flow from the atria to the ventricles, but not in the other direction:
    - Tricuspid valve – a valve with three flaps, known as cusps, that allows blood to flow from the right atrium into the right ventricle
    - Mitral valve – a two-cusp valve that allows blood to flow from the left atrium into the left ventricle.

- Two semilunar valves, which are shaped like half-moons and have three cusps each. They allow blood to flow out of the heart from the ventricles to the two exiting arteries, the pulmonary artery and the aorta, but not in the other direction:
    - Pulmonary valve – a valve with three cusps that allows blood to flow from the right ventricle to the lungs through the pulmonary artery

- Aortic valve – a three-cusp valve that allows blood to flow from the left ventricle into the aorta and then to the rest of the body.

What happens during the cardiac cycle as the heart beats

Deoxygenated blood is returned to the heart via two main veins, called the superior vena cava and the inferior vena cava. The superior vena cava brings blood back from the upper part of the body and the inferior vena cava from the lower parts of the body. These veins pour the deoxygenated blood into the right atrium.

The pulmonary veins carry oxygen-rich blood back from the lungs to the left atrium and are the only veins to carry oxygenated blood.

Let us look now at the two main phases in the heart cycle, or in each heartbeat, which are called diastole and systole:

Diastole

During this phase the ventricles are both relaxed. Blood is passed from the two atria into the ventricles via the two atrioventricular valves. The right atrium pumps blood into the right ventricle through the tricuspid valve and the left atrium pumps blood into the left ventricle through the mitral valve. As the pressure inside the ventricles rises, it will cause the atrioventricular valves to close, preventing blood from flowing back into the atria. This is the end of diastole.

Systole

During this phase, which refers to the contraction of the heart muscle in the ventricles, the right ventricle starts to pump momentarily before the left ventricle. This causes blood to be pumped into the pulmonary artery to the lungs, where it is oxygenated. The left ventricle then contracts, pumping blood into the aorta and out to the rest of the body. The ventricles then collapse and seal all of the valves, so that no blood can get in from either the atria or from backward flow from the pulmonary artery or aorta. This then triggers the atria to fill again.

Figure 1: The circulation

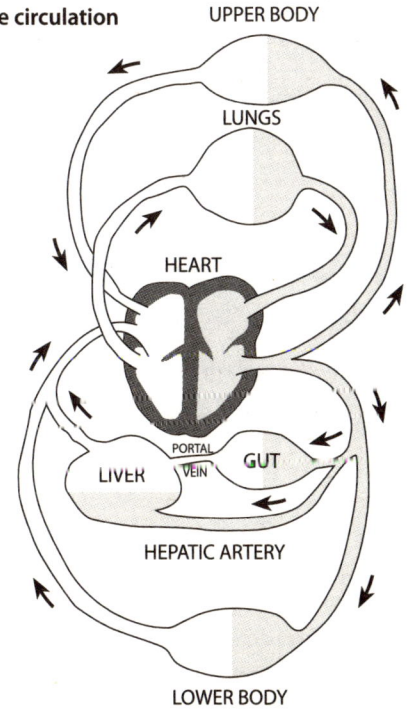

The conducting system of the heart

The heart beats every minute of your life. It does this by virtue of an electrical conducting system within the heart muscles.

There is a natural pacemaker located in the right atrium. It is called the sinoatrial node. It causes a wave of electrical activity to spread out over the muscle of both atria, causing them to contract and pump blood into the ventricles.

The wave of activity then causes another point in the very middle of the heart muscle, called the atrioventricular (or AV) node, to trigger another impulse that spreads down the wall between the ventricles, along the right and left 'bundles of His' to the Purkinje system (see box below), causing the ventricles to contract to pump blood out to the lungs from the right ventricle and to the body from the left ventricle.

It is this wave of electrical activity that we measure when an electrocardiogram (ECG) is done. We shall consider it in more detail in Chapter 11.

> **THE 'BUNDLES OF HIS' AND THE PURKINJE SYSTEM**
>
> The 'bundles of His' are specialised conducting tissues that descend in bundles from the atrioventricular node down through the ventricle walls, one on the right and one on the left, to reach the Purkinje tissues, a network of specialised conducting tissues which permeate throughout the rest of the ventricle walls.
>
> The Purkinje system was described in 1845 by Johannes E. Purkinje, a Bohemian anatomist, and the 'bundles of His' were described by the German cardiologist and anatomist Wilhelm His Jr in 1893.

Figure 2: The electrical conducting system of the heart and the ECG which measures the electrical activity of the heart

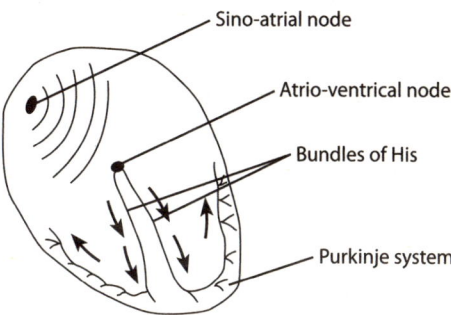

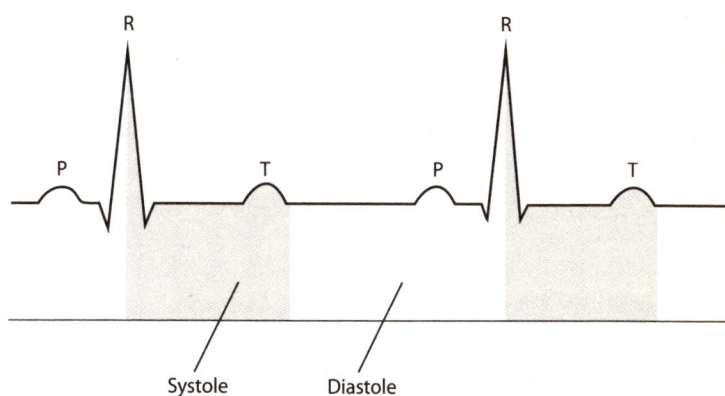

KEY POINTS ABOUT THE BLOOD VESSELS

There are four types of blood vessel: arteries, arterioles, capillaries and veins.
- Arteries carry blood away from the heart to the organs and tissues, and veins carry it back to the heart.

- Arteries generally carry oxygenated blood to the tissues to nourish them.
- Arterioles are the very smallest arteries, which link up with capillaries.
- Capillaries are tiny thread-like blood vessels that join the arterial circulation to the venous circulation. They feed the tissues.
- Veins carry deoxygenated blood back to the heart, in order for it to be pumped to the lungs to receive more oxygen.

The aorta is the main artery of the body. It comes out direct from the heart and supplies all of the other arteries of the systemic circulation with oxygen-rich blood. The point to note is that arteries carry blood away from the heart. All of the arteries of the systemic circulation carry oxygenated blood from the left ventricle.

The pulmonary artery is an exception, since it carries deoxygenated blood from the right ventricle to the lungs, where the blood is oxygenated and then returned to the heart by the pulmonary veins, which are the only veins to carry oxygenated blood.

The lung tissue itself is supplied by the bronchial arteries, which are derived from the thoracic aorta, that is from the aorta as it passes down through the thorax (chest).

The blood

There are about 8–10 pints of blood in the average adult and that blood makes up roughly 9 per cent of our body weight. It is composed of:

- A fluid called plasma, which is 91 per cent water and 9 per cent solids and other contents: proteins, salts, digested products, waste products, oxygen, carbon dioxide gases,[i] hormones, enzymes and various messenger chemicals.

- Blood cells:
    - Red blood cells, which carry the oxygen.
    - White blood cells, of various types, which fight infection and protect the body.
    - Platelets, which clump together to produce clots to plug any breaches in blood vessels.

The blood supply to the heart

Most people find it surprising to know that although the heart pumps blood around the body, it still needs to have its own blood supply. If it doesn't get oxygen from blood, pain will be felt and the individual will experience angina (more of which later). Worse still, if part of the heart is deprived completely of oxygen-rich blood for a mere 5–10 minutes, then that part of the heart muscle may die.

The reason for having its own blood supply is that the heart is made up of specific muscle tissue called the myocardium. This has to be given its oxygen – and all the other nutrients that the blood supplies – in exactly the same way as every other tissue of the body: it has to receive it from the arterioles that run through it. And they in turn have to be supplied by their own arteries.

---

[i] Oxygen is carried in the blood in two ways, either bound to haemoglobin in the red blood cells (the vast majority is carried this way), or dissolved in the plasma. Carbon dioxide is carried in the blood in three ways, either carried by haemoglobin or dissolved in plasma or in the form of bicarbonate ions.

This is similar to the lungs, which also have to have their own blood supply, quite apart from the blood that is pumped through them to pick up oxygen.

The heart – a majestic organ

The coronary arteries are the blood vessels that supply the heart direct. The name comes from the Latin *coronarius*, meaning crown. They are essentially a crown or garland of blood vessels that supply the heart muscle direct.

There are two main coronary arteries, the left coronary artery and the right coronary artery. They both arise from the main blood vessel, the aorta, soon after it leaves the heart from the left ventricle. Each coronary artery supplies a different part of the heart with oxygenated blood:

Figure 3: The coronary arteries

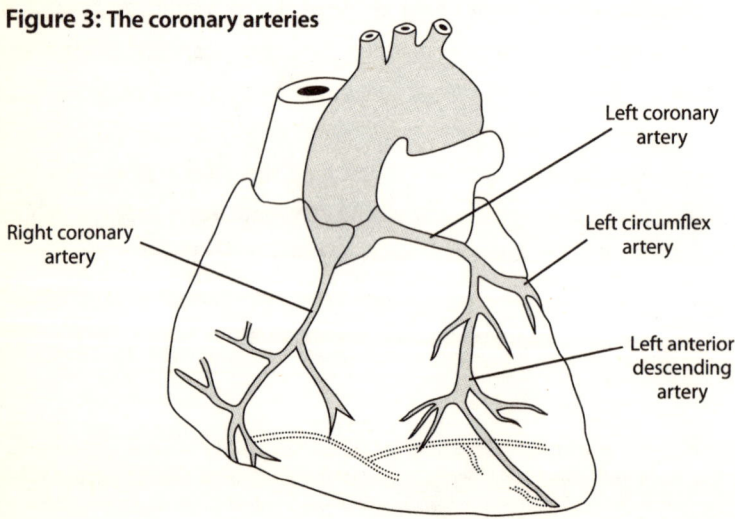

- Right coronary artery – supplies oxygenated blood to the walls of the right atrium, the right ventricle, the lower 25 per cent of the left ventricle, and the back of the septum (the wall between the two sides of the heart).

- Left coronary artery – divides the oxygenated blood it carries into two vessels:

    - Left anterior descending artery – supplies the front and bottom of the left ventricle and the front of the septum. Essentially, this is the front of the heart.
    - Left circumflex artery – supplies blood to the walls of the left atrium, and the side and back of the left ventricle.

Chapter 2

The different types of cardiovascular disease

Cardiovascular disease (CVD) is an umbrella label for all of the diseases and disorders of the heart and circulation.

> **KEY POINTS**
> - Over 2.7 million people are affected by chronic heart disease in the UK.
> - Cardiovascular disease causes over 88,000 deaths in the UK each year.
> - Coronary heart disease, also known as ischaemic heart disease, is the commonest cause of death in the UK (about 82,000 each year).
> - Over 124,000 people have a heart attack each year.
> - About two million people in the UK suffer from angina.
> - Strokes are the third-commonest cause of death (causing 11 per cent of deaths in England and Wales), after ischaemic heart disease and cancer of the lung.
> - There are approximately 110,000 first strokes in the UK per year.
> - There are approximately 30,000 recurrent strokes in the UK per year.

Let's get the names right

Already you may have noticed that there are a number of terms used which can be quite confusing. This book is mainly going to deal with coronary heart disease and conditions of the heart that may arise from it, as well as conditions that may predispose to coronary heart disease. It is important to understand exactly what we mean, so it is worth spending a little time to clarify the different terms.

Cardiovascular disease

This is the umbrella term for all diseases of the heart and the circulation.

There are four main types of cardiovascular disease:

- Heart disease
- Stroke
- Peripheral artery disease
- Aortic artery disease.

Heart disease

This relates to all conditions that affect the heart itself.
There are four main types of heart disease:

- Coronary heart disease or CHD
- Congenital heart disease
- Valvular heart disease
- Cardiomyopathy.

Coronary heart disease

This is, in terms of morbidity and mortality, by far the commonest. It is the cause of angina and heart attacks, and is the subject of the majority of this book.

It is caused when the coronary arteries of the heart (which supply the heart muscle with oxygen) get blocked up by atheroma (fatty plaques), a process referred to as arteriosclerosis or hardening of the arteries. We will consider this in the next chapter.

It may not cause any symptoms at all until the restricted blood flow gets so bad that the heart muscle starts to experience cramp and the pain of an angina attack will be felt. Or until a thrombus (blood clot) blocks one of the coronary arteries, causing a heart attack (the medical term for which is 'myocardial infarction').

> A couple of confusing terms used in coronary heart disease
>
> - Coronary artery disease (CAD) – this refers to the disease process in which the coronary arteries become blocked.
> - Ischaemic heart disease (IHD) – this refers to the state when the heart muscle is deprived of oxygen. Ischaemia comes from the Greek *iskhein*, meaning 'to restrict'. It is sometimes used instead of 'coronary heart disease'.

THE DIFFERENT TYPES OF CARDIOVASCULAR DISEASE

KEY POINTS

The main consequences of coronary heart disease are all caused by restriction of blood flow along the coronary arteries to the heart:

- *Angina* – sudden chest pain on exertion, eased by rest. This is the commonest manifestation of CHD.

- *Heart attack, also known as a myocardial infarction or MI* – occurs when a coronary artery is blocked and part of the heart muscle is damaged or dies. A heart attack can be life-threatening. There are a number of other terms used, which we shall consider in the relevant chapter.

- *Heart failure* – when a reduced blood supply to the heart affects the muscle to the extent that the heart's ability to function as a pump is impaired. This can cause breathlessness or accumulation of fluid in the feet, ankles and legs.

- *Arrhythmias or irregular beating of the heart* – there are several types of irregularity, some of which can be life-threatening if they lead to cardiac arrest, when the heart stops beating.

LATIN OR GREEK

About 90–95 per cent of all medical terms are based on Latin or Greek.[6] Most of the anatomical terms that you will find in this book are of Latin origin. That is because Latin terminology comes from antiquity and later from the Renaissance, when Latin was still used as the language of science and medicine. The titles of the books by Andreas Vesalius and William Harvey, which I talked about in the last chapter, are examples of this.

> By contrast, most of the terms referring to diseases and pathological processes are derived from the Greek language. This dates back to the knowledge and skills of the early Greek physicians.
>
> For those who are interested, I will indicate the origins of terms as we go through the book. Essentially, think Latin for anatomy, and Greek for conditions and processes.

Congenital heart disease

This refers to a problem or abnormality of the heart that is present from birth. It occurs in about one in every 150 births. Over half of these do not cause any restriction in the life of the individual or can be easily corrected by surgery after birth.

Others are quite severe, since they may seriously incapacitate the heart's ability to work as a pump.

Infections contracted by the mother during pregnancy, such as rubella (German measles), can cause congenital heart disorders, as can some drugs taken during pregnancy – thalidomide, used as a sleeping tablet and anti-nausea drug for pregnant women in the late 1950s and early 1960s, was later associated with congenital malformation of babies' limbs. It was discontinued for such uses and as a more general result there is a reluctance to prescribe any drugs during pregnancy unless absolutely necessary. Holes in the heart or between the chambers of the heart, or abnormalities of the heart valves, are among the sort of problems that can occur through illness or absorption of drugs during pregnancy.

Valvular heart disease

There are four valves in the heart, all of which prevent blood from flowing in one or other direction.

Problems can occur if a valve gets narrowed, the medical term for which is 'stenosis'. This may restrict the flow of blood between chambers inside the heart, or valves can become incompetent or start to leak, so that blood flows backwards. Both types of valvular disease can cause their own problems, which we shall consider in the chapter on valvular heart disease.

Cardiomyopathy

This is the name given to disease of the heart muscle. It may be a disorder that is genetic, in that it runs in families.

There are three types of cardiomyopathy, which we shall consider in more detail in Chapter 9:

- Hypertrophic cardiomyopathy (HCM)
- Dilated cardiomyopathy (DCM)
- Arrhythmogenic right ventricular cardiomyopathy (ARVC)

Stroke

A stroke is the name given to a brain attack in which an area of the brain is deprived of its blood supply. The blood supplies the brain with oxygen and nutrients, including glucose. If the blood supply is cut off to a part of the brain then the delicate brain cells will start to become damaged and quickly die off. This takes place within a mere six minutes, so time is of the essence.

It is important to appreciate that **a stroke is always a serious event and should be treated as a medical emergency**. Permanent damage to the brain, or even death, can occur.

The blood supply to the brain was discovered by Dr Thomas Willis in the mid-seventeenth century. Essentially, the two internal carotid arteries in the front of the neck pass up into the skull and form a ring with vessels from the Basilar artery, which is itself formed from two vertebral arteries which pass up the back of the neck into the back of the skull. This ring is called the Circle of Willis. It is located underneath the brain.

Smaller arteries then branch off from it and travel upwards to supply very specific parts of the brain.

When someone has a stroke it may be possible, on the basis of the clinical examination, to deduce which part of the brain has been affected:

- Anterior cerebral arteries supply the front of the brain and the motor and sensory areas for the lower part of the body. A blocked anterior cerebral artery may cause paralysis and sensory deficit on the opposite side of the body from the hips down. There can also be incontinence of the bowel or the bladder. Since it supplies the frontal area some personality change can occur.

- Middle cerebral arteries supply the areas involved in speech, swallowing and language function. They supply a large part of the brain, including the corpus striatum, which is involved

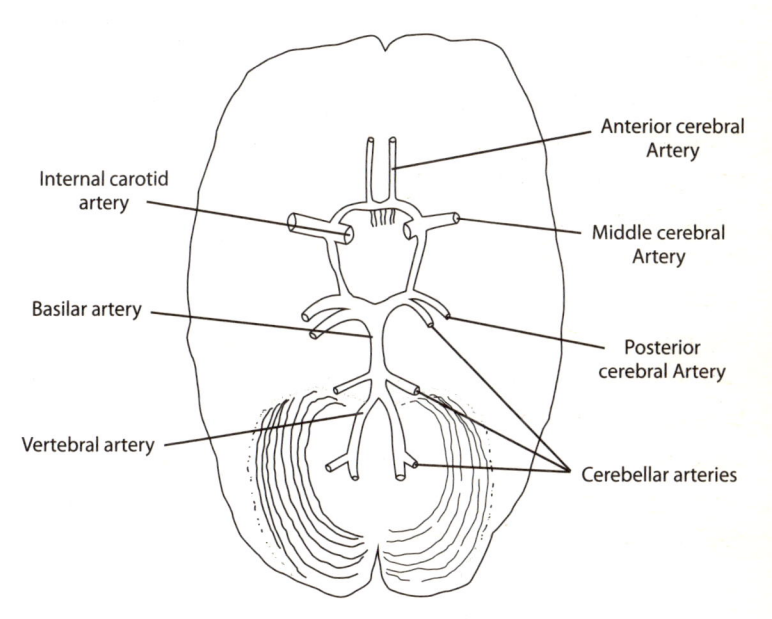

Figure 4: The blood supply of the brain

- Anterior cerebral Artery
- Internal carotid artery
- Middle cerebral Artery
- Basilar artery
- Posterior cerebral Artery
- Vertebral artery
- Cerebellar arteries

in regulating our movements, and so a blockage can result in a wide variety of problems. A stroke affecting the middle cerebral arteries can also cause a specific visual defect called hemianopsia, in which half of the visual field is impaired in each eye.

- Posterior cerebral arteries supply a lot of the hind part of the brain. Since this area has a large part to play in vision, there can be a wide variety of visual problems associated with blockages.

- Cerebellar arteries supply the cerebellum, so blockages are often associated with ataxia, or balance and coordination problems.

In the case of a stroke, the blood supply to the brain can be affected in one of two ways:

Ischaemia

This means that a blockage occurs in a blood vessel. Generally this is the result of cholesterol plaques building up inside the vessel. Essentially, it comes about as a result of a hardening of the arteries, which is explained more fully in Chapter 3.

There are two ways that an ischaemic stroke can occur:

- If a plaque on a brain blood vessel ruptures, a clot rapidly forms about the damaged area. If this is large enough to block the flow of blood then the part of the brain supplied by that blood vessel may be damaged.

- If a clot forms in another part of the body and flows along the circulation to lodge in a narrow part of an artery supplying the brain. This also produces ischaemia. Such a clot is called an embolus.

Ischaemia accounts for 80 per cent of strokes.

Haemorrhage

This is when a bleed into the brain itself occurs when a blood vessel bursts. It accounts for the other 20 per cent of strokes.

Peripheral artery disease

Peripheral artery disease means disease of the arterial system to the limbs. For practical purposes, it refers to the narrowing of the blood supply to the lower limbs. It is also sometimes known as occlusive disease, or as peripheral vascular disease.

> **KEY POINTS**
>
> The pathological process involved in peripheral artery disease is exactly the same as with coronary heart disease. That is, it is arteriosclerosis (hardening of the arteries) affecting the arteries of the lower limbs.
>
> - The classic symptom is called 'intermittent claudication'. This is pain developing in the calf muscles or sometimes in the buttocks after walking a certain distance. This distance is variable. Some people only get it after walking a few hundred yards, others as little as 30 yards. Stopping to rest eases the pain.
> - If peripheral artery disease is present, then the individual is likely to also have coronary artery disease and cerebrovascular disease (disease of the blood supply to the brain). Indeed, half will have a history of either a previous stroke or a heart attack.

Aortic artery disease

The aorta is the main blood vessel of the systemic circulation. It comes out of the left ventricle of the heart and gives off branches to the head and neck and to the four limbs. It is a huge blood vessel, as thick as a garden hose. It runs from the heart, through the chest and down through the abdomen.

The pathological process is the same as it is for coronary heart disease and, in fact, aortic artery disease is really a type of peripheral artery disease.

The most common problem with the aorta is the development of an aortic aneurysm. This is a bulging of the aorta, caused by a weakening of its wall. It is potentially dangerous because blood clots can form on damaged internal walls and be carried to another part of the body where they may obstruct a smaller blood vessel with catastrophic results. Or they can rupture, again with potentially fatal consequence.

KEY POINTS

There are two main types of aortic aneurysm, depending on which part of the body they develop in:

- Thoracic aortic aneurysms (TAA) – these occur in the arch of the aorta and account for 25 per cent of aortic aneurysms.
- Abdominal aortic aneurysms (AAA) – these occur in the abdominal aorta, just below the renal arteries that supply the kidneys. They account for the other 75 per cent of aortic aneurysms.

Figure 5: Aneurysms of the aorta – top shows an aortic aneurysm and bottom shows abdominal aortic aneurysm

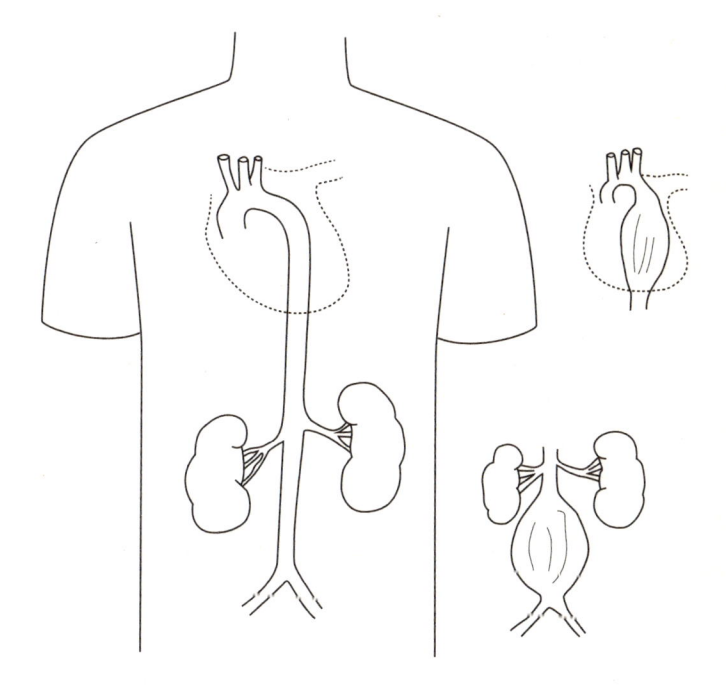

Chapter 3

Hardening of the arteries

The basic problem that causes many of the disorders of the cardiovascular system is hardening of the arteries.

Arteriosclerosis and atherosclerosis

The medical name for hardening of the arteries is arteriosclerosis. It is a normal part of ageing as continuous pressure makes the vessel walls harder and stiffer.

Atherosclerosis is actually a specific type of arteriosclerosis that causes problems in coronary heart disease (CHD), cerebrovascular disease (CVD) and peripheral artery disease (PAD). The word comes from the Latinised version of the Greek *athero*, meaning gruel or porridge, and the Greek *sclerosis*, meaning hardening. This image of producing a hardened porridge-like interior to the arteries is not far from what actually happens – the lining of the blood vessels accumulates a patchy covering that is grainy, rough and sticky, just like gruel or porridge.

KEY POINTS

- Atherosclerosis is the basic problem that causes CHD, CVD and PAD.
- Atherosclerosis is the process in which atheroma is laid down in arteries
- Atheroma may restrict blood flow.
- The rupture of an atheroma plaque can cause a clot to form inside a blood vessel.

The anatomical structure of the arteries

If we look at a cross section through an artery we can delineate three layers.

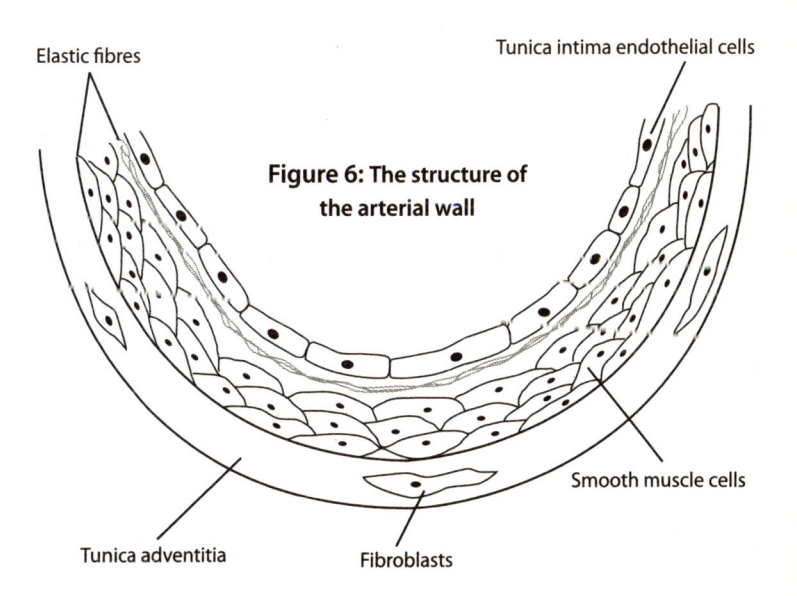

Figure 6: The structure of the arterial wall

Elastic fibres
Tunica intima endothelial cells
Smooth muscle cells
Tunica adventitia
Fibroblasts

Tunica intima – this is the innermost layer, which consists of flat cells that are arranged rather like paving stones to produce a smooth surface. The cells are called endothelial cells and are stuck together by a glue of polysaccharides, which are long carbohydrate molecules made up of repeating units of sugars. Underneath, they have a connective coating of elastic tissue called the internal elastic lamina.

Tunica media – this is the middle and thickest layer of an artery wall. It is essentially elastic connective tissue and smooth muscle cells. It is bound by another layer of elastic tissue called the external elastic lamina.

Tunica externa (or *tunica adventitia*) – this is connective tissue that contains nerves and tiny capillaries, which supply the cells of the vessel. This is the thickest layer in veins.

The space inside the blood vessel, through which blood flows, is called the lumen.

The pathological process – what actually happens

The process of hardening of the arteries is a slow, gradual build-up over many years. It goes on without the individual being aware of any problem, until the blood flow is so reduced that symptoms appear because the heart is called upon to pump more blood, or until a clot and its associated blockage of the artery in question occurs.

> **KEY POINT**
>
> Hypertension or high blood pressure is one of the causes of atherosclerosis, because sustained high pressure in the artery wall can damage it, leading to the build-up of atheroma.

Atheroma plaques, also called fatty plaques, develop inside the artery wall, which will have an effect not unlike the silting up of a riverbed. As a result, blood flow to the tissues being supplied is reduced.

These plaques can encircle the whole lining of the artery or may be quite eccentric as an isolated blob on a part of the internal artery wall.

How the atheroma fatty plaques build up

The plaque is the result of a process that starts when the endothelial cells get damaged. A number of factors that can cause this sort of damage include:

- Toxic chemicals from tobacco.
- Oxidised low-density lipoprotein (bad cholesterol).
- Infectious agents.
- Metabolic products, such as homocysteine (a type of amino acid that in high levels may cause inflammation inside blood vessels, leading to the development of atheroma plaques).

When endothelial cells are damaged there is a reduction in the production of various defensive chemicals and hormones, whose role it is to maintain the integrity of the cells.

Circulating white blood cells (leucocytes) are attracted to the damaged area and bind to the endothelial cells. Then they migrate through the endothelial lining to lie underneath it. They tend to become transformed into macrophages, which are large cells whose function is to engulf and digest debris and microbial invaders. The name comes from the Greek *makros,* meaning 'big,' and *phagein,* meaning 'eat'. They are 'big eaters'. What they then do is scavenge and absorb low-density lipoprotein cholesterol (the bad cholesterol) and become foam cells. These are characteristic of atheroma plaques.

The earliest lesions are called fatty streaks and they simply consist of these foam cells. Gradually they absorb calcium and they develop a fibrous coating, as smooth muscle cells get transformed into fibre. By this stage the atheroma is producing a lump that will start to intrude into the lumen of the artery.

It gradually becomes more organised and develops a fibrous cap. The interior of the atheroma plaque consists of foam cells, cholesterol crystals and calcium. It really deserves the porridge-like description of atheroma. While this fibrous cap remains intact, however, blood flows over it and symptoms may not occur.

Lots of atheroma lesions can develop along the course of an artery, the net effect being to narrow it along a significant length, thereby reducing the flow of blood through it. If this happens in the coronary arteries that supply the heart, then angina may be the result.

Atheroma is most likely to build up at curves in the arteries, or where branches and tributaries are thrown off from a main trunk.

All of this process has the effect of altering the structure of the artery wall, so that it becomes much less elastic, much more rigid and much more vulnerable. It becomes hardened.

Figure 7: The build-up of artheroma

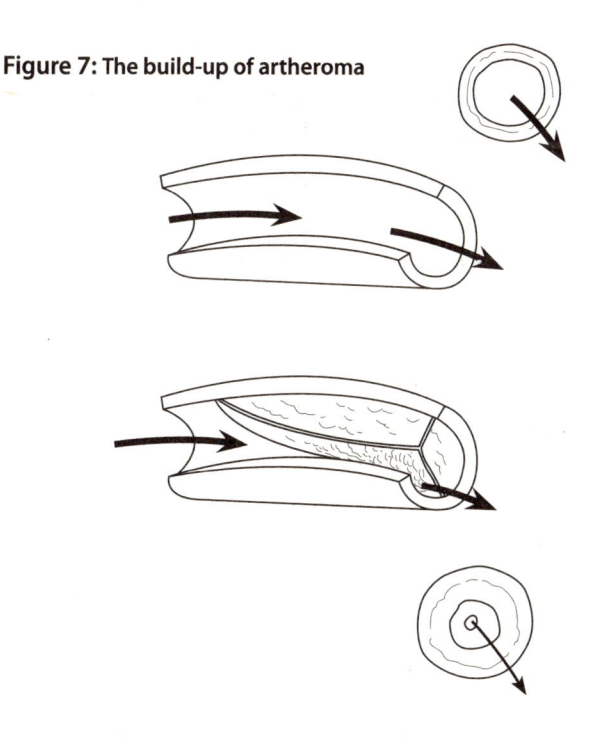

It can take 30 years or more to develop significant atherosclerosis. The danger point is reached when an atheromatous plaque ulcerates, like a miniature volcano, to cause thrombus formation, as described below, possibly with a cataclysmic result. Such ruptures of plaques can occur from forty years of age and upwards.

Thrombus formation

In atherosclerosis a plaque or atheroma can suddenly rupture, whereupon a cascade reaction occurs which causes a clot to form over the ruptured plaque in order to seal the damaged wall. It is essentially a normal body reaction to self-seal a damaged area. The problem is that the cells that are being mobilised to do so, and which fulfil the function that they are designed for, have no awareness that they could be forming a clot that could be catastrophic for the whole organism.

An atheroma plaque can rupture if its pulp becomes necrotic, which means the cells inside it die and it just becomes too big to be contained by the fibrous capsule.

As long as the inner walls of the vessel remain smooth, then the blood will flow. However, if that layer is disrupted by the *rupture of a plaque*, then messenger chemicals will alert blood cells, which, as we have seen, will move to the area to form a clot to seal off the damaged part of the vessel. Platelets will accumulate and a fibrous structure like a spider's web will be formed to catch more and more cells to help seal the damage. This is called a thrombus, and the process of thrombus formation is called thrombosis.

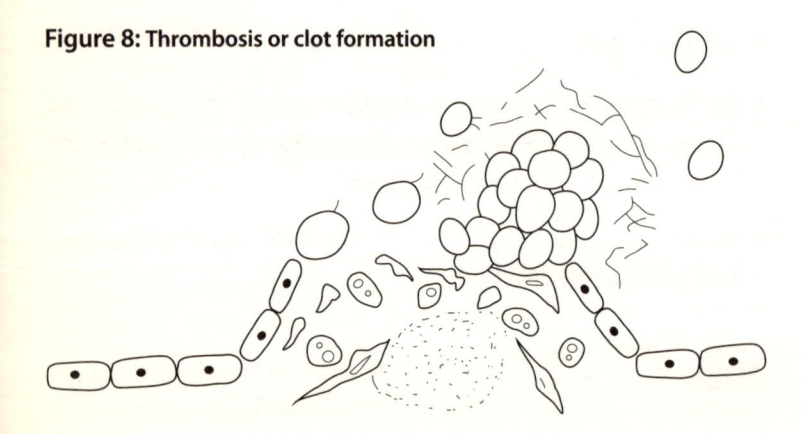

Figure 8: Thrombosis or clot formation

If the coronary artery is very narrow and the thrombus becomes big enough to block off the flow of blood, then a heart attack is likely. The part of the heart that is supplied by that artery will die.

The consequences of atherosclerosis

The pathological process now having been outlined, we are in a position to consider the various clinical conditions that may result from atherosclerosis affecting the coronary arteries (as we have seen, the process of atherosclerosis causes the arteries to become harder and less elastic, and causes the insides to get progressively blocked up, a bit like the furring up of water pipes).

And we can now see how it underlies many of the cardiovascular diseases that were outlined in Chapter 2:

- Coronary heart disease – by blocking the coronary arteries of the heart.

- Stroke – by affecting the arteries that supply the brain.

- Aortic artery disease – when bulges, or aneurysms, develop. The danger is that the aneurysm wall is weakened and that it could burst, with catastrophic consequences.

- Peripheral artery disease – by blocking the arteries that carry blood to the limbs.

> **KEY POINTS**
>
> The coronary arteries can be affected by atherosclerosis in three ways:
>
> - They can become progressively hardened and narrowed.
> - They can get completely blocked.
> - The arterial wall can become stretched, resulting in an aneurysm.

Blockage of arteries causes two types of problem

If an artery is only partially blocked and therefore still allows a flow of blood to the tissues, then it may not cause any symptoms. Symptoms may occur when a critical point is reached, or if the body is asked to do extra work necessitating more oxygen. The impaired circulation cannot provide this and the tissues become deprived of oxygen.

Ischaemia

The tissues of the body all need oxygen to function and to survive. Whenever the blood supply is inadequate, the tissue is said to have become ischaemic. Nerve tissue, especially brain cells, cannot survive more than a few seconds without oxygen.

The myocardium, the muscle of the heart, cannot sustain ischaemia for long, either. The consequence is pain. This is the mechanism of pain in angina pectoris or in a heart attack. This is why the term ischaemic heart disease is often used interchangeably with coronary heart disease.

Infarction

When deprived of oxygen beyond a critical point, cells start to die. This is called infarction. The infarction of heart muscle may lead to instant cardiac failure and sudden death.

If death does not occur then the myocardium will undergo various pathological changes. It basically results in the muscle cells being replaced by fibrous connective tissue, to produce a scar. This is less elastic than heart muscle and is potentially weaker. It is not 'functioning', so it shows up as non-activity on the ECG. This produces the changes that allow doctors to make their diagnoses.

Myocardial infarction is the name we give to a heart attack. It means that some of the heart muscle (myocardium) has been damaged and has therefore died. In some heart attacks the damage is to the full thickness of the heart muscle and in others it is only partial. This is important, as we shall consider later in Chapter 13.

Anatomical consequences

- Just as certain points in a plumbing system may be more prone to furring up, so too are certain parts of the circulatory system more prone to develop atheroma. It is common in the coronary arteries, but more so in the left coronary artery.

- The commonest site of a myocardial infarction is the anterior (front) two-thirds of the left ventricle wall between the ventricles, especially at the apex of the heart (left anterior descending artery territory).

- Infarcts only rarely occur in the atria.

Chapter 4

Hypertension (high blood pressure)

Hardening of the arteries is not the only cause of cardiovascular disease. High blood pressure, which is also known as hypertension, can also do so. Indeed, hypertension can itself be a cause of atherosclerosis, because sustained high pressure in the arteries can cause damage to the arterial walls, which is how atherosclerosis can begin.

> **KEY POINT**
>
> Raised blood pressure is caused by the smallest arterial blood vessels, the arterioles, reducing in calibre. Even a small restriction can produce a marked increase in pressure.

What is hypertension?

This is actually not an easy thing to define and experts have argued about it for years. The best working definition of it is that it is a chronic condition, in which the levels of blood pressure are such that there is a significant risk to health, and that treatment can reduce the risk.

It is sensible for all adults to have their blood pressure recorded at least once every five years, since it is an insidious condition that can creep up on an individual without them having any symptoms whatsoever. If it is found to be borderline in terms of hypertension, then it needs to be checked every year.

> **KEY POINTS**
> - People often assume that headaches will be the first symptom of hypertension, but more often than not, it is a symptomless condition. The only way you can find out if you have it is by having your blood pressure measured.
> - Uncontrolled high blood pressure is the biggest reversible risk factor for several cardiovascular conditions, including stroke and heart attack.

The dangers of hypertension

The longer the blood pressure is raised, the greater the risk of damage to blood vessels. It can affect all sizes of arteries, from the very smallest arterioles to the medium-sized coronary arteries and even the large aorta. Let us look at the various ways in which hypertension can affect the heart and/or the circulatory system:

Atherosclerosis

As already mentioned above, high blood pressure can be a direct contributor to atherosclerosis.

Angina pectoris

This is pain in the chest on exertion, caused by ischaemia. It occurs when atherosclerosis impedes the flow of blood significantly, so that when the person exerts him or herself the heart is unable to supply enough oxygen-rich blood to the heart muscle, which develops cramp pain. We shall consider this in more detail in Chapter 5.

Myocardial infarction

Because hypertension can promote atherosclerosis, it significantly increases the risk of having a myocardial infarction. Therefore the prevention of high blood pressure is well worthwhile in terms of reducing one's future risk of heart attack.

Heart failure

Long-standing hypertension can damage the heart muscle, causing the heart to become stiff, which in turn can result in difficulty filling the ventricle with blood. It can also make the muscle weak, causing a back-pressure effect on the lungs. Fluid then collects in the lungs and the person concerned becomes breathless. We shall see in Chapter 6 that a weak heart and a stiff heart can both produce heart failure, and whichever one is the case will have implications for the treatment required.

Atrial fibrillation and arrhythmias

Hypertension can cause the heart to become uncoordinated, in that the chambers may not function in harmony. Atrial fibrillation (an abnormal heart rate) may be the result, which is a risk factor for stroke.

Stroke

Because hypertension increases atherosclerosis, which, as we know, narrows and weakens the arteries, the increased pressure within the arteries can also cause the rupture of a brain blood vessel, thereby producing a stroke (a brain attack caused by disruption to its blood supply). A stroke can either be the result of a blockage (as in a heart attack) or a haemorrhage of a brain blood vessel.

Dementia

The increased pressure in the cerebral circulation can increase the damage caused by atherosclerosis and can predispose to dementia. We know so little about this condition and have so few ways of preventing it, but controlling blood pressure is certainly one of them.

Kidney damage

The kidneys are involved in the control of normal blood pressure. Paradoxically, they are very much at risk in the event of sustained high blood pressure. Kidney function can be impaired and this can lead to increased risk of a heart attack or stroke (or to kidney failure itself).

Peripheral artery disease

As we have seen, the arteries to the lower limbs can develop atherosclerosis and become progressively narrower, obstructing the flow of blood to those extremities and, if severe enough, causing intermittent claudication (pain in the calf muscles while walking). Raised blood pressure can worsen this condition by causing further damage to the lining of the blood vessels and increasing the atherosclerosis.

Aortic aneurysm

High blood pressure can cause the weakened (from atherosclerosis) wall of the aorta to bulge, creating an aneurysm which can burst and produce haemorrhaging that requires emergency surgical treatment.

> **KEY POINTS**
> - Most aortic aneurysms do not rupture.
> - They occur in one in 25 males over 65 years.
> - One in 100,000 people have a ruptured aortic aneurysm every year.

Eye damage

The delicate blood vessels in the retinae of the eyes can be damaged by hypertension. Blood vessels can get narrowed and/or thickened and may haemorrhage. Eye examination should be a regular part of the management of hypertension.

> **KEY POINTS**
> - Hypertension affects over ten million people in the UK.
> - In the United Kingdom, the prevalence of hypertension has been estimated to be 42 per cent in people aged 35 to 64.
> - A health survey for England in 2003 showed that 31.7 per cent of men and 29.5 per cent of women in the adult UK population have hypertension.
> - Hypertension directly causes half of all the strokes and heart attacks in the UK.[7]

What is blood pressure?

Blood pressure is the force of blood against the walls of arteries, and is recorded as two numbers. Firstly, the systolic pressure, which represents the pressure attained as the heart beats. Secondly, the diastolic pressure, which represents the pressure in the circulation as the heart relaxes between beats. The measurement is written with the systolic figure on top and the diastolic number on the bottom, thus 120/80. These numbers each represent the recorded pressure in mmHg. This means mm of mercury, which is the standard means of measuring pressure. It is for historical reasons that we measure it like this, as we shall see in the next section.

It is currently recommended that a level of 140/85 or less is the level that should be aimed at in treatment. To put the risk into figures, each rise of 2 mmHg of systolic pressure increases the risk of mortality from heart disease by 7 per cent, and of mortality from stroke by 10 per cent. Keeping the blood pressure controlled, therefore, is the single most important thing to do to reduce the risk of heart disease or stroke.

The discovery of blood pressure[8]

Nowadays, the taking of a person's blood pressure is regarded as one of the basic parts of a physical examination. It is interesting that the first experiments upon it were done not by a medical practitioner, but by a Church of England priest, the Reverend Stephen Hales, in the eighteenth century.

The Reverend Stephen Hales (1677–1761) was intensely interested in science and he had ample time to pursue his interest. He conducted 25 experiments on several dogs, three horses, a sheep and a doe, and published his findings in his *Statical Essays* in 1733. He deduced that the maximum pressure of the blood was reached at the end of a cardiac contraction, and that this would give an idea about cardiac output. He also deduced that the lowest pressure would be a measure of the resistance to flow and that this would occur during the relaxation of the heart.

These were extremely important findings, but it was not until a century later that any practical means of measuring blood pressure could be developed. Even then the methods of measuring were invasive, involving the insertion of tubes (cannulation) into arteries, so they were of no use in clinical medicine. It then took another 50 years before a non-invasive, practical method was devised. In 1896 Scipione Riva-Rocci invented the mercury-based sphygmomanometer (more of which in a moment) and this was subsequently refined by Heinrich Von Recklinghausen. In neither of these versions was a stethoscope used. Indeed, the stethoscope was still a relatively new instrument and it did not occur to anyone that there were useful sounds that could provide information about blood pressure.

The Korotkoff sounds

A Russian doctor, Nikolai Korotkoff (1874–1918) wrote a thesis about his use of the stethoscope to measure blood pressure in 1910. It was entitled *Experiments for determining the strength of the arterial collaterals*. In this thesis he outlined the method of taking blood pressure that has been used right up until the present day.

This involved applying a cuff attached to the sphygmomanometer and listening with a stethoscope over the brachial artery at the elbow. The cuff is inflated until the radial pulse is no longer felt. The reason for doing this is to collapse the vessel, by making the pressure in the cuff greater than in the blood vessel. Then the cuff is slowly deflated. A series of different sounds will be heard. The first one is the noise of blood flowing at maximum blood pressure. Then other sounds are heard, having significance in relation to the cardiac cycle, although we need not go into the technicalities in detail here. The point at which the sounds disappear is the important one, as this represents the minimum blood pressure.

Modern sphygmomanometers

Nowadays electronic sphygmomanometers are used, since they are extremely accurate at detecting blood flow. They have by and large replaced the traditional method of listening with a stethoscope, although a lot of doctors still trust to their ears and the traditional method of listening to the Korotkoff sounds.

Yet it has to be said that when a human being is involved in taking a reading, there can be bias inherent in the measurement. Some doctors and nurses have more acute hearing than others, so they might hear the sounds earlier, resulting in higher readings being recorded by some of them.

The important thing to ensure is that sphygmomanometers are properly calibrated. In the UK, the British Hypertension Society offers guidelines on the devices that have been 'standardised'.

It is also possible to get home-recorders, but it should be noted that the ones that measure at the fingers or the wrists might be quite inaccurate. The pressure should be taken at the same level as the heart, which means with a cuff around the upper arm.

The causes of hypertension

About 95 per cent of cases of hypertension are not associated with any underlying cause. That is, they are referred to as essential hypertension, or primary hypertension.

The other 5 per cent are called secondary hypertension, and may be caused by one of the following:

Renal disease

There are several renal (kidney) disorders that may cause hypertension:

- *Diabetic nephropathy* – a kidney disease that complicates diabetes.

- *Renal artery stenosis* – narrowing of the renal artery, the main arterial supply to the kidney. Your doctor may listen to your back to determine if a bruit, the sound of turbulence in the flow of blood through the artery, is audible.

- *Glomerulonephritis* – the name for a number of conditions that cause inflammation in the glomerulus, a sensitive part of the kidney.

- *Chronic pyelonephritis* – persistent infection of the kidney, or kidneys.

- *Polycystic kidneys* – this is a genetic condition causing multiple cysts on the kidneys.

Endocrine disorders

The endocrine system is the name given to those glands of the body that produce the hormones (chemical messengers) that regulate the various functions of the body. They are ductless glands, which means that they do not have a duct (tube) that allows their secretions to flow out, so that they directly pass their hormones into the bloodstream or the lymphatic system that flows through them. Endocrine disorders include the following:

- *Cushing's syndrome* – this is a disorder that is caused by too much cortisol in the body. It is associated with weight gain, thinning skin, stretch marks, and fat deposits on the face that give it a moon-shaped appearance. It can be caused as a drug side effect from too many steroids given for other conditions, or by a tumour of the pituitary gland (situated at the base of the brain) pumping out too much ACTH (adrenocorticotropic hormone), which then stimulates the adrenal glands to produce excess amounts of cortisol.

- *Conn's syndrome* – this is an adrenal disease in which the adrenal gland produces excess aldosterone hormone. It is also known as *primary aldosteronism*.

- *Hyperparathyroidism* – this is a disorder of the parathyroid glands, of which there are four embedded in the substance of the thyroid gland in the neck. Excess parathyroid hormone can cause hypertension (as well as kidney stones, problems with calcium metabolism, abdominal pain and bone pain).

- *Phaeochromocytoma* – this is a rare tumour of the adrenal gland, which tends to cause paroxysmal (sudden or violent) hypertension and arrhythmias, which occur when the tumour pumps out catecholamines – adrenaline and noradrenaline.

- *Acromegaly* – this is a condition in which too much growth hormone is produced. It tends to become apparent in people of 30 to 50 years of age. Coarsening of the features, increase in teeth spacing and increase in foot size are indications that growth hormone is at work. It is associated with an increase in blood pressure and sometimes with cardiomyopathy (heart muscle disease).

Drugs

Some 'recreational' drugs, like amphetamines, cocaine and ecstasy (MDMA), can push blood pressure up. So too can some medicinal drugs, such as non-steroidal anti-inflammatory drugs (NSAIDs), steroids, some antidepressants (e.g. trimipramine and venlafaxine), and the oral contraceptive pill.

Even cold remedies that may be bought over the counter can contain decongestants that exert their effect by narrowing blood vessels. As this may increase the blood pressure, they should be avoided in people with known hypertension. Decongestants that can elevate the blood pressure include: phenylephrine, pseudoephedrine and ephedrine.

Alcohol

A little alcohol seems to have a beneficial effect on health, but too much is hazardous. It can certainly cause the blood pressure to rise.

Coarctation of the aorta

This is a congenital condition in which the aorta is pinched and constricted shortly after it leaves the heart. It may cause raised blood pressure and/or different pressures in the two arms.

Diet

Too much salt taken in the diet can increase blood pressure. So too can too much liquorice or too much coffee (four or more cups of coffee a day may elevate the blood pressure).

Pregnancy and pre-eclampsia

The blood pressure can go up during pregnancy, but for most women this is not a problem. In pre-eclampsia, a condition caused by narrowing of the blood vessels in the placenta, the blood pressure may rise dangerously high. It affects between 5 and 8 per cent of pregnancies. In the UK, severe cases cause the deaths of up to ten women and up to a thousand babies a year.

It is important to have all of the above conditions excluded whenever hypertension is diagnosed, since they may need to be treated per se and may even result in a cure of the hypertension. With essential hypertension, on the other hand, there is no cure, but there are many effective treatments, as we shall see in Chapter 16.

The way the body controls blood pressure

It is quite important to understand how the body controls blood pressure, since it gives us a way of understanding how we can control it with drugs. It will also help us understand later in the book how drugs can help in coronary heart disease.

Homeostasis

This is the name that we give to the body's ability to control its internal workings and inner environment. This all takes place involuntarily, meaning that we do not have to think about it. It just takes place. The autonomic nervous system is one of the means by which this occurs, and there are two main components to it:

- Sympathetic nervous system – which prepares us for 'fight or flight' (and which we will look at in more detail shortly)
- Parasympathetic nervous system – which controls the functions that allow us to 'rest and digest'.

The sympathetic and parasympathetic systems by and large produce opposite effects, yet complement each other. You can think of the sympathetic nervous system's role as preparing your body for an emergency, while the parasympathetic nervous system restores normal functioning after the emergency has passed. The sympathetic nervous system is the one that is most essential in terms of blood pressure control.

The endocrine system includes all of the so-called 'ductless glands', which produce hormones. These are chemical messengers, which exert an effect on metabolism and the way in which other organs operate. Examples are the pituitary gland, the thyroid, the pancreas and the adrenal glands.

A specific hormonal system is also relevant in blood pressure control. It is the complex-sounding, but very elegant, renin-angiotensin-aldosterone system (which we will return to shortly).

The sympathetic nervous system

This consists of a double chain of ganglia that are present on either side of the spinal cord, in the thoracic and lumbar areas of the body. (Ganglia are bundles of nerve tissues containing nerve cell bodies, which act like signal boxes to relay impulses to different nerves.) They are connected to the central nervous system and the organs of the body via nerve fibres, and they work by releasing the neurotransmitters adrenaline and noradrenaline. They in turn cause adrenergic receptors in the target organs to produce the sympathetic effects. These are:

- Eye – the pupil is dilated

- Heart – the rate is increased and the force of each heartbeat, each contraction, is increased

- Lungs – the bronchioles, the small air tubes, are dilated

- Blood vessels – the arterioles, the very smallest arteries, are constricted

- Sweat glands are activated to allow for heat control

- Digestion is reduced and the peristalsis (intestinal movements that push food along the alimentary tract) is reduced

- Kidney – stimulated to produce the hormone renin (more of which later).

One can see how these mechanisms are useful in an emergency situation, or at a time of danger. If the sympathetic system is not subsequently shut off, however, its continued effects can result in raised blood pressure.

> **KEY POINTS**
>
> The sympathetic nervous system:
>
> - Constricts arterioles
> - Speeds up the heart and increases the strength of contractions
> - Causes the kidneys to produce renin.

You may wonder why the blood vessels should be constricted. Well, that is one of the body's mechanisms to control blood pressure. If the pressure is too low, perhaps as a result of a haemorrhage or fluid loss, then the sympathetic nervous system will crank up the pressure in order to ensure that the brain receives its required amount of blood.

The parasympathetic nervous system by contrast has a craniosacral outflow, meaning that it is connected to the central nervous system by the cranial nerves (which come direct from the brain, rather than from the spinal cord) and the sacral part of the system (the lower part of the spine and back of the pelvis). It operates with the neurotransmitter acetylcholine, reversing the effect of the sympathetic nervous system and increasing salivation, tear production, digestion, urinary function and excretion.

So the sympathetic and parasympathetic nervous systems complement each other, but control different parts of our functioning. When all is well, the parasympathetic system will switch off and reverse the effects of the sympathetic system. But if it does not, the ongoing sympathetic activity will keep the blood pressure raised. And that can produce hypertension.

The renin-angiotensin-aldosterone system

I said that this is an elegant system. I think you will see what I mean as I run through the way the different organs of the body are involved in it.

As mentioned above, if blood pressure drops, then the sympathetic nervous system immediately kicks in and raises the pressure by constricting the arterioles. This is just a temporary matter, however, and has to be boosted by a longer-term effect. This is where the renin-angiotensin-aldosterone system comes in. This system involves the kidneys, the liver and the lungs.

We have seen from the sympathetic nervous system's effect on the kidney that the hormone renin is released into the bloodstream. Renin is an enzyme, which plays an important role in controlling blood pressure.

When blood pressure drops, it causes the liver to produce a protein molecule called angiotensinogen. It then breaks it down into another protein called angiotensin I.

When the renin from the kidneys reaches the liver, it stimulates the liver to break down more and more angiotensinogen into angiotensin I.

The lungs then release an angiotensin-converting enzyme, commonly known as ACE, which causes the angiotensin I to be broken down into a far more active protein called angiotensin II. This has a vasoconstrictor effect (meaning it causes blood vessels to constrict and narrow) throughout the whole circulation, causing blood pressure to rise.

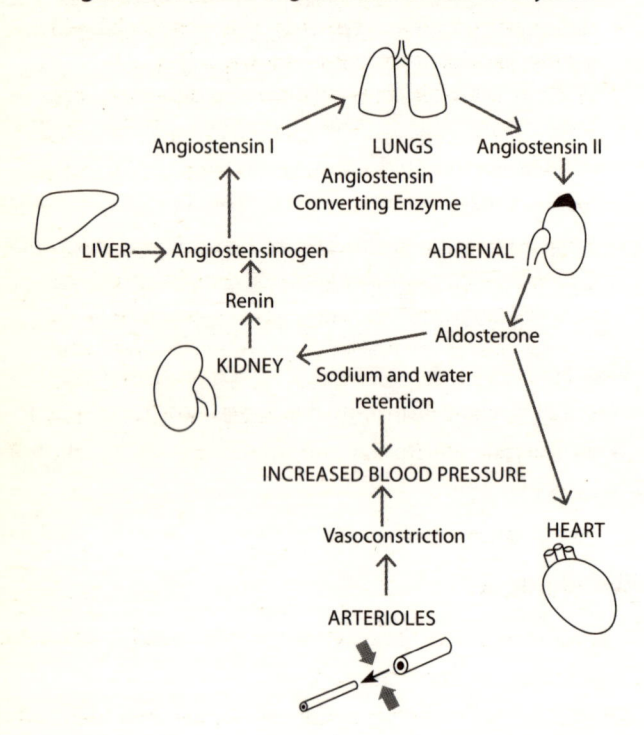

Figure 9: The renin-angiostensin-aldosterone system

The angiotensin II also causes the two adrenal glands, one of which sits on top of each kidney, to secrete a hormone called aldosterone. This hormone then works on the kidneys to cause sodium and water retention, which in turn maintain the required blood pressure increase.

> **KEY POINTS**
>
> - The sympathetic nervous system and the renin-angiotensin-aldosterone system combine to regulate blood pressure, i.e. to restore to it to the right level if anything causes it to drop.
>
> - People with hypertension do not have excessive amounts of hormones in their body – their systems are just more reactive to those hormones.
>
> - In the treatment of hypertension and heart failure, we use various strategies aimed at interfering with the sympathetic nervous and renin-angiotensin-aldosterone systems. For example, we use ACE inhibitor drugs to prevent the production of angiotensin II from angiotensin I, or alpha-blocking drugs to reduce sympathetic activity on blood vessels and allow them to relax and dilate.

Calcium channels

There is another important mechanism that we need to consider. It is to do with calcium concentrations.

The arterioles have smooth muscle cells inside their walls, which operate to dilate or constrict them. In the presence of calcium within the smooth muscle cells the muscle fibres contract. This causes the arteriole to constrict.

Calcium enters the cells through calcium channels. For some reason the calcium levels in these cells is raised in people with hypertension, as compared with those with low blood pressure. The exact mechanism by which this happens is not clear, but the effect is to elevate and sustain blood pressure.

We have various antihypertensive treatments that act as calcium channel blockers, which we shall look at in more detail later.

Chapter 5

How coronary heart disease manifests itself

Although we think of coronary heart disease as being a problem of modern life, it was in fact a condition that afflicted the ancients. At the beginning of the twentieth century Sir Marc Ruffer, a physician at the Faculty of Medicine at Cairo University, conducted a study of arteries in a number of Egyptian mummies. He described the marked presence of atherosclerosis in several of them, including the royal mummy of Merneptah (reigned 1213–1203 BC), the supposed pharaoh of the Exodus. He had gained the throne at about the age of 60, after all of his elder brothers predeceased him. His mummy showed extensive arthritis and arteriosclerosis. It is likely that this was the cause of his death, rather than drowning in the Red Sea.[9]

The different presentations

In medicine we refer to the 'presentation' of a problem. This means the way in which a condition tends to present itself to the patient and to the doctor. Thus, although we know that the underlying problem in diabetes mellitus is a problem with blood sugar, the symptoms that are presented are likely to be increased thirst and increased passage of urine. Yet not all patients with diabetes present in this classic way. Others may present with an infection of the bladder, or an infection of the skin, or an increased tendency towards thrush. This is because diabetes predisposes the person to an increased risk of infections.

Similarly, although several patients may have coronary heart disease, it may present in different ways. We looked at those ways fleetingly in Chapter 2. Now we can look at them in a little more detail to understand more about how they manifest themselves.

- *Angina* – sudden chest pain on exertion, eased by rest. This is the commonest manifestation of CHD.

- *Heart attack, also known as a myocardial infarction or MI* – occurs when a coronary artery is blocked and part of the heart muscle is damaged or dies. A heart attack can be life threatening.

- *Heart failure* – when the blood supply to the heart affects the muscle to the extent that the heart's ability to function as a pump is impaired. This can cause breathlessness or accumulation of fluid in the feet, ankles and legs.

- *Arrhythmias (irregular beating of the heart)* – there are several types of irregularity, some of which can be life threatening if they lead to cardiac arrest, when the heart stops beating. Atrial fibrillation is one of the commonest of these arrhythmias and carries the risk of inducing a stroke.

Chest pain – the commonest symptom

This is undoubtedly the commonest symptom and it is due to ischaemia in the myocardium (the muscle of the heart) caused by an inadequate supply of oxygen.

> **KEY POINT**
>
> The tissues of the body all need oxygen in order to function and survive. Whenever the blood supply is inadequate, the tissue is said to have become ischaemic.

We tend to differentiate the chest pain of coronary heart disease into two main types:

- *Angina pectoris* – which is ischaemia but without infarction. It classically comes on exertion, is predictable, and is short-lasting.

- *Acute coronary syndrome* – this is chest pain that is less predictable and more severe. It can be either angina that is getting worse, when it is called 'unstable angina', or it can be a heart attack.

Angina pectoris

This is chest pain that is typically brought on by exertion and relieved by rest. The name comes from the Latin 'angina', meaning 'choking pain' and 'pectoris', meaning 'chest'. Cases of it have been described for centuries, yet the first good clinical description was given by the eighteenth-century English physician Dr William Heberden, in his book *Commentaries on the History and Cure of Diseases*. He had studied nearly a hundred people with the condition and found that most cases occurred in men over the age of 50. Only three women were seen. His description of it is regarded as one of the classics of medicine. Here is a part of what he wrote:

> But there is a disorder of the breast marked with strong and peculiar symptoms…
>
> They who are affected with it are seized while they are walking (more especially if it be uphill, and soon after eating) with a painful and most disagreeable sensation in the breast, which seems as if it would extinguish life, if it were to increase or to continue; but the moment they stand still, all this uneasiness vanishes.
>
> In all other respects, the patients are, at the beginning of this disorder, perfectly well, and in particular have no shortage of breath, from which it is totally different. The pain is sometimes situated in the upper part, sometimes in the middle, sometimes at the bottom of the os sterni[ii], and often more inclined to the left than to the right side. It likewise very frequently extends from the breast to the middle of the left arm.
>
> Males are more liable to this disease, especially such as have past their fiftieth year.

The usual presentation of angina

Described in the language of today, angina is a severe chest pain that is experienced on exertion, such as lifting or going uphill. It usually only lasts two or three minutes, and it generally dissipates with rest. It starts in the left side of the chest and radiates into the left arm or

---

[ii] Os sterni – the sternum or breast bone

up into the neck and throat, and is often described as a pressing or crushing pain in the chest. It may or may not be associated with an increase in perspiration and a clamminess.

> **KEY POINT**
>
> A sudden attack of chest pain, or chest pain coming on exertion and easing off on resting, should be considered to be angina until proven otherwise. A medical opinion is needed straight away. Your doctor may refer you to a fast-track angina clinic.

Management of angina

Diagnosis is the first thing, and we shall consider the diagnostic tests that are employed when we look at dealing with heart disease in Part Two of the book.

Drug treatment can be very effective, to the extent that the condition is often completely controllable, as we shall also see in Part Two.

> **TYPES OF ANGINA**
>
> It is usual to classify angina into four different types, according to when it occurs and its relationship to exertion:
>
> - **Stable angina** – this is the classic description just given, when the conditions that bring it on are predictable.
> - **Unstable angina** – this may cause pain on the slightest of exertions, or even when resting. It can occur even after the very first attack of chest pain and be the diagnosis arrived at after assessment in hospital. It is more serious than stable angina.

- **Crescendo angina** – this refers to rapidly increasing attacks of angina. It indicates worsening of an underlying problem with the coronary arteries.
- **Decubitus angina** – this is a variant whereby angina is provoked when the person lies flat, and which is usually indicative of heart failure. Someone with this condition may only be able to sleep propped up on several pillows because, if they lie too flat, the deterioration in blood flow may bring on the angina attack.

Acute coronary syndrome

As mentioned above, this is the name given by doctors to cover unstable angina and myocardial infarction (heart attack). It is the term used when the patient is admitted to hospital with acute chest pain (so we shall look at it again in Part Two of the book when we cover what happens in hospital).

KEY POINTS

Each year 114,000 people are admitted to hospital with acute coronary syndrome. The type of acute coronary syndrome they suffer from is determined by:

- The location of the blockage
- The length of time that blood flow is blocked
- The amount of heart muscle damage that has occurred.

Unstable angina

In stable angina the chest pain is predictable. The individual knows what can be done to prevent an angina attack without having to experience it, and what sort of situation or activity will provoke it. With unstable angina, the attacks of angina become less predictable and can occur more frequently and with less exertion. It can even wake the person from sleep, which is always an alarming thing. If any of these symptoms occur, medical aid should be summoned urgently.

In unstable angina the blood flow through the coronary arteries is severely impaired, yet enough of a trickle is getting through to supply some oxygen to the heart muscle, so it does not infarct or die.

The important thing to appreciate is that this is a worsening situation that may reflect that the underlying coronary heart disease is getting worse. The narrowing of the coronary arteries may be getting more severe and it is possible that a heart attack could be the next part of the process.

> **KEY POINTS**
> - Fifteen per cent of people with unstable angina will suffer a myocardial infarction in the following month.
> - If angina attacks are occurring at rest, this indicates the need for hospitalisation.
> - If an angina attack lasts more than 20 minutes, this too indicates the need for admission to hospital.

Myocardial infarction (or heart attack)

This manifests itself as a severe chest pain, often described as the worst pain imaginable. It is vice-like, and occurs in the same distribution as angina, i.e. on the left side of the body. It may come out of the blue, without any previous history of angina. Quite simply, it can come on if a blockage in one of the coronary arteries suddenly arises from a clot (thrombosis).

Not all heart attacks produce this debilitating pain, however, and about 20 per cent of heart attacks are silent – that is to say, the person is not even aware that they have had one, perhaps attributing the symptoms to a bout of indigestion. This is more likely to be the case in the elderly.

There are essentially two types of heart attack, depending upon the amount of damage that occurs to the heart muscle. They are called ST elevation myocardial infarction (STEMI) and non-ST elevation myocardial infarction (NSTEMI). The ST refers to the ST parts of the wave found on the ECG (see Figure 2 in Chapter 1). In STEMI there is obvious elevation of the ST segment of the ECG, whereas in NSTEMI there is either no alteration or a temporary alteration in the ST segment in the ECG.

- STEMI – the arterial supply to part of the heart muscles is completely blocked off.
- NSTEMI – the arterial supply is only partially blocked off, so only part of the heart muscle is damaged.

It is important to differentiate between them, since they require different types of treatment. Since STEMI is due to sudden blockage by a clot, the mainstay of treatment is thrombolytic (clot-busting) treatment. Primary angioplasty may also be used. NSTEMI, on the other hand, is due to an unstable clot (clumping of platelets) so its mainstay treatment is antiplatelet drugs or anticoagulants.

> **KEY POINTS**
>
> A heart attack is always serious:
>
> - About 240,000 people have a heart attack in England and Wales every year.
> - 50 per cent of those who die from a heart attack do so within the first hour.
> - Death is commonly due to an abnormal rhythm of the heart being provoked when the conducting tissue of the heart is affected.
> - The risk of death declines hour by hour.
> - Emergency treatment is essential, including the immediate use of aspirin and access to a defibrillator if necessary.
> - Most cases of acute coronary syndrome occur in the over-50s.

As we shall see in Chapter 12, an exact diagnosis depends on the findings of an ECG test, blood tests to assess myocardial damage, and the histories of the event and patient. Certain symptoms may develop as a direct result of the heart attack itself, and each will need to be treated in its own way:

Complications of myocardial infarction

- *Heart failure* – of which there may be variants. We shall look at this in the next chapter.

- *(New) heart murmur* – which could indicate a hole developing inside the heart between the ventricles, or the rupture of a muscle operating a heart valve. Cardiac surgery may be necessary to repair the damage.

- *Pericarditis* – inflammation of the pericardium, the sac that contains the heart. Drugs to reduce the inflammation may need to be given.

- *Post-infarction angina* – which will require investigation.

- *Irregularities of the heart rhythm* – which can be acute and therefore life-threatening, or chronic and requiring investigation and stabilisation.

- *Fever* – this may be part of the process, or it could indicate an infection.

- *Ventricular aneurysm* – after a myocardial infarction the scar tissue formed may be weak and the result would be a ballooning out of the ventricular wall. This can occur in the first few days or weeks after a heart attack. It will tend to be associated with heart failure and cardiac surgery may be needed.

Chapter 6

Heart failure

Heart failure is a complex matter. It sounds frightening, but it does not necessarily mean that the heart is going to stop or that the failure is irreversible.

Essentially it means that the heart is failing to adequately fulfil its functions. It is not pumping enough blood around the body to the organs and tissues at the right pressure. As a result, it can produce a variety of symptoms. For example, fluid can accumulate in the lungs (causing breathlessness), ankles may start to swell and the person concerned generally feels fatigued for much of the time.

With medical treatment, however, the chances are that heart failure can be addressed and improved.

> **KEY POINTS**
>
> - Heart failure is the fastest-growing cardiovascular condition[10]
> - Heart failure affects 2–3 per cent of the overall population of the UK
> - The prevalence rises with age and affects 10–20 per cent of the over-70s.

The many causes of heart failure

Heart failure is not the same thing as heart disease. Heart disease may be a cause of heart failure, but so too can several other conditions:

- *Hypertension* – high blood pressure can throw a strain on the heart and lead to heart failure.

- *Coronary heart disease* – the commonest cause of heart failure. About 70 per cent of heart failure sufferers have coronary heart disease.

- *Myocardial infarction* – may be an immediate cause of heart failure.

- *Cardiomyopathy* – because it causes weakness of the heart muscle.

- *Arrhythmias, especially atrial fibrillation* – by causing abnormal rhythm or incoordination of the heart, the heart may not fill adequately, and so eventually it will fail.

- *Valvular disease* – this causes about 10 per cent of heart-failure cases.

- *Alcoholic cardiomyopathy* – alcohol can affect the heart muscle by weakening it, or it can have a toxic effect that leads to irregular beating of the heart.

- *Drug side effects* – so-called recreational drugs like cocaine may cause heart failure. So too can some medications as a side effect, e.g. various drugs used in chemotherapy.

- Radiotherapy can in some cases cause heart failure.

- *Post-viral impact* – some viral illnesses may seem to have got better, but may in fact have weakened the heart and thereby caused heart failure to develop.

- *Anaemia* – this can tip the heart into failure, by causing it to work harder to supply more blood to the tissues, since the anaemia makes the blood less effective in carrying oxygen.

- *Thyroid overactivity* – this can overwork the heart by speeding it up.

- *Pulmonary hypertension* – high pressure in the lungs can cause a backward pressure effect on the heart, thereby tipping it into failure.

- *Connective tissue disease*, such as systemic lupus erythematosus – may cause heart failure through a direct effect on the heart or on the lungs.

- *Nutritional deficiencies* – not common in this country, but beriberi, a condition caused by deficiency of vitamin B1 (thiamine), can cause heart failure.

- *Sarcoidosis (enlarged lymph nodes) and amyloidosis (unwanted insoluble proteins)* – these are infiltrative conditions that can both cause heart failure.

- *Congenital heart disease* – for example, a hole in the heart may significantly affect the haemodynamics (blood flow) of the heart.

The importance of diagnosing not just heart failure, but the cause of that heart failure, is clearly important, since treatment of the underlying condition may cause a marked improvement. If the problem is a valvular heart disorder, then surgical treatment of the valve may be curative.

The different forms of heart failure

There are many different causes of heart failure, as seen above. Many people have more than one cause, which is why it can be such a complex condition. There are predominantly three ways in which they cause the heart to fail:

- They weaken the heart
- They make the heart too stiff
- They make the heart beat in an uncoordinated manner.

Let us look more closely at how these three damaging conditions might arise:

Left ventricular systolic dysfunction (LVSD) – this is a weak heart. The left ventricle, which pumps blood around the body, has become too weak and fails to pump enough blood out during the heartbeat. Hence it is called systolic dysfunction. Common causes of LVSD are:

- Coronary heart disease
- Heart attacks
- Cardiomyopathy.

Diastolic heart failure – this is a stiff heart, resulting in difficulty in filling with blood, because the ventricle can't relax enough to fill up. It is sometimes also called 'heart failure with preserved ejection fraction' (HFpEF). The ejection fraction is the term used to describe how much blood is pumped out by the ventricle during the heartbeat. It is expressed as a percentage. A normal ejection fraction is 50–60 per cent. Below 40 per cent is abnormal.

Common causes are:

- Old age, especially in women
- Hypertension.

Heart failure due to valvular disease – this is caused by the mechanical problem of leaking heart valves, causing the heart to do extra work. Or it can be stiff valves, which again cause the heart to overwork.

High output failure – this is when the heart is made to work extra hard as a result of certain conditions, e.g. thyrotoxicosis (overactive thyroid gland), anaemia, long-standing hypertension, Paget's disease (a bone disorder) and beriberi.

Acute or chronic onset of heart failure

Heart failure can come on extremely rapidly, such as after a myocardial infarction, or very gradually. If it comes on rapidly (acutely) then the body has no opportunity to establish compensatory mechanisms, the result being that it develops severe breathlessness and accumulation of fluid in the lungs. Acute heart failure can occur after a heart attack, or after an arrhythmia.

Chronic heart failure can build up over a long time and the body gradually develops mechanisms to compensate. For example, with long-standing hypertension the myocardium will undergo hypertrophy, which means the muscle will actually become larger. The heart can cope for a while, but it does so inefficiently and eventually it will be followed by compensatory dilatation of the ventricle, which will reduce its function, and failure becomes manifest.

Right or left heart failure

Heart failure can affect the left, the right or both sides of the heart. (As we have seen, the right side receives oxygen-depleted blood from the rest of the body and pumps it out to be replenished by the lungs, whereas the left side receives oxygen-rich blood from the lungs and pumps it out to the rest of the body.)

Left-sided failure or LVF (left ventricular failure) is more common and results in insufficient oxygen-rich blood being pumped out. Instead, it backs up into the left atrium and pressure then builds up in the circulation to the lungs (called pulmonary venous congestion or pulmonary oedema). The person feels tired because of lack of oxygen, and breathless due to fluid build-up in the lungs.

> **KEY POINT**
>
> Acute LVF is a medical emergency because the patient literally fights for breath. It may often be a presentation with a myocardial infarction.

Symptoms with left-sided failure

- Shortness of breath
- Reduced mobility

- Breathlessness at rest
- Breathlessness gets worse on lying down in bed at night, so person has to use extra pillows
- A dry cough may develop that doesn't go away
- Fatigue
- Muscle weakness
- Weight loss, in advanced cases.

Right-sided failure causes the congestion to back up from the right side of the heart to the rest of the body. This is called systemic venous congestion. It causes congestion in the liver and will cause the liver to enlarge (this is called 'hepatomegaly'). There will also be the development of swollen ankles, which, if very severe and long-lasting, can extend right up the legs to the abdomen.

Symptoms with right-sided failure

- Swelling (oedema) in the legs.
- Dry skin and ulceration of the skin on the lower part of the legs because of pressure from inside the tissue. This can cause flaking.
- There may be an eczema-type rash on the legs, which can be complicated by venous leg ulcers. These can be very difficult to heal.
- Possible accumulation of fluid in the abdominal cavity (ascites).
- Swelling and congestion of internal organs, especially the liver.

Congestive heart failure – this is the name given when both right and left failure are present.

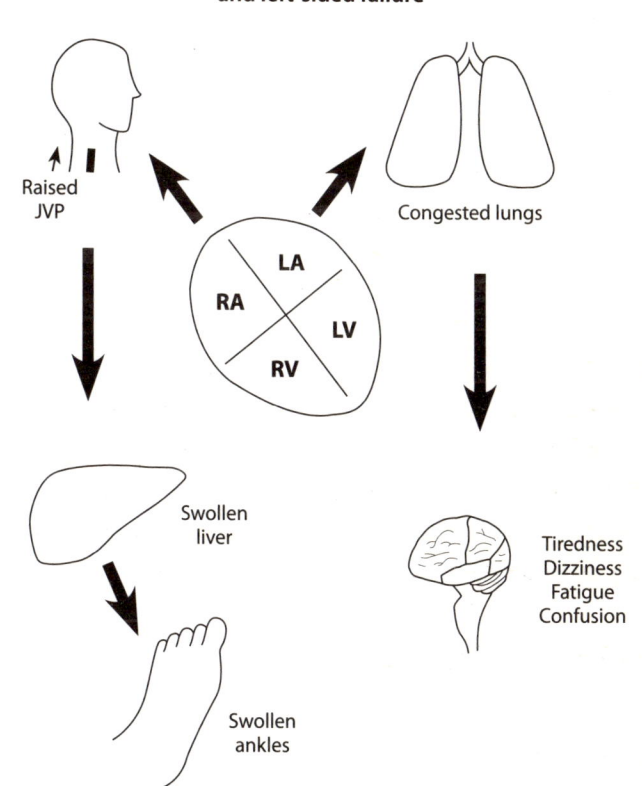

Figure 10: The back pressure effects of right-sided failure and left-sided failure

Self-regulating mechanisms sometimes go over the top

The body has an incredible array of mechanisms, which regulate our metabolism and the way that our organs work. Some of these are under nervous control and others are biochemical.

As we saw in Chapter 4, there are two mechanisms that are very important in the way that the body maintains blood pressure, the sympathetic nervous system and the renin-angiotensin-aldosterone system. They are important for doctors to understand, in order to develop treatments. They are also highly significant in heart failure, since when the heart starts to fail, they are both stimulated into greater activity. Unfortunately, their attempts to do what they usually do act against the body to produce some of the symptoms of heart failure. But, as with blood pressure, it is important to understand how these mechanisms come into play, since we can target treatments to minimise their effects and thereby help the heart failure.

Sympathetic nervous system

As the heart failure progresses, the sympathetic nervous system is activated. This causes vasoconstriction of small blood vessels and tends to predispose to irregular heart rhythms and to sodium retention. It will also cause an increase in renin release (renin is the enzyme that has a crucial role in blood pressure control, as discussed in Chapter 4).

Renin-angiotensin-aldosterone system

You will recall from Chapter 4 that this is a hormonal system that operates to maintain blood pressure, but its role in the event of heart failure is counterproductive, because it tends to make it worse.

The renin release catalyses the breakdown of angiotensinogen to angiotensin I, which is then broken down by the angiotensin converting enzyme (ACE) into angiotensin II. This is the most powerful vasoconstrictor (constrictor of blood vessels) in the body, and it has the effect of increasing both the cardiac preload (the amount of blood in the ventricles at the end of diastole) and the cardiac afterload (the resistance that the ventricles must overcome in order to circulate the blood).

Effectively the angiotensin II causes more blood to be squeezed into the heart during filling in diastole, but also acts to increase the resistance in the systemic circulation, which makes the ventricle have to work harder. The tendency will be for the ventricle to dilate, which makes it less efficient.

The angiotensin II also has the effect of increasing aldosterone release from the adrenal gland. This will cause more sodium and fluid retention, which will accumulate in the lungs in the case of left ventricular failure, and in the organs and extremities in the case of right ventricular failure.

Figure 11: Pre-load and after-load. Pre-load is like a hose filling the ventricle and after-load is like a tap restricting outflow

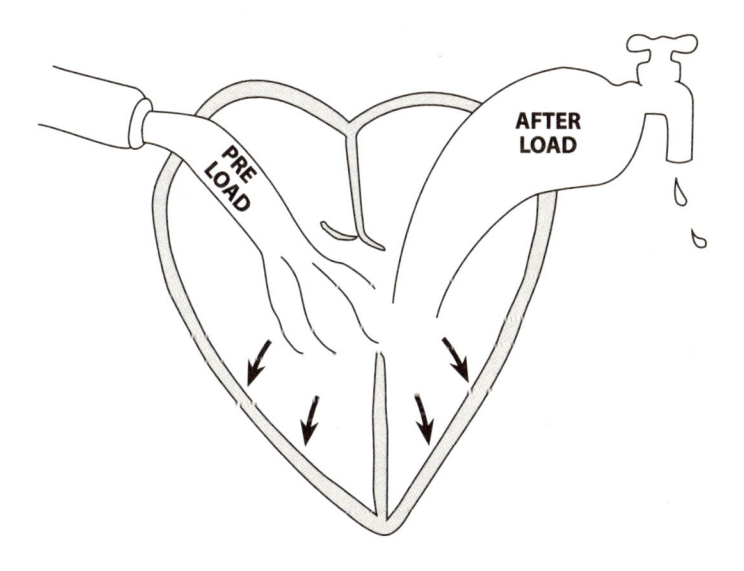

UNDERSTANDING AND DEALING WITH HEART DISEASE

Figure 12: Some of the sites of action of drugs used in the treatment of heart failure and hypertension

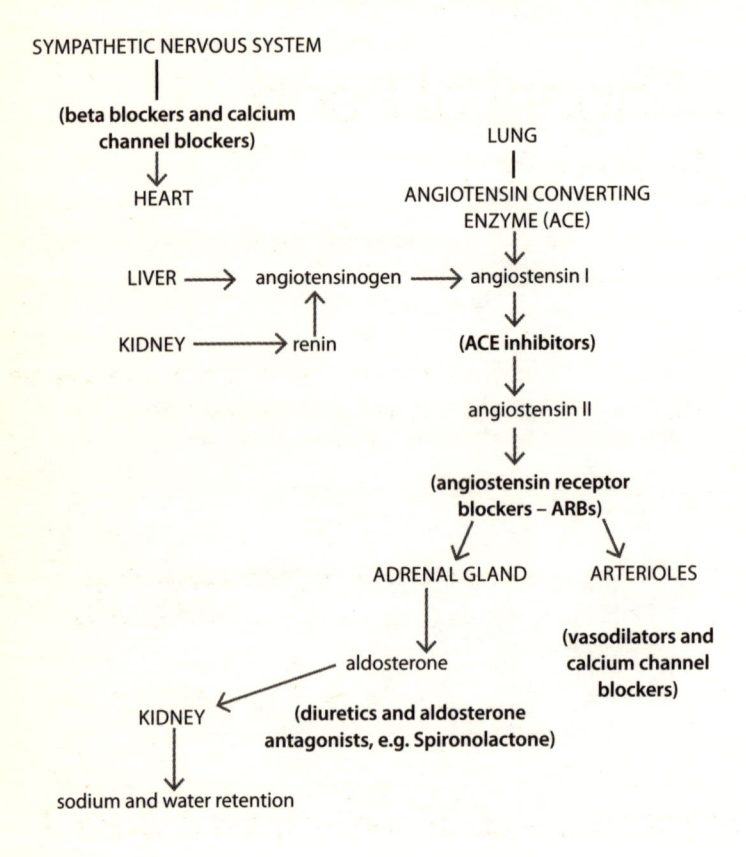

SYMPATHETIC NERVOUS SYSTEM
|
(beta blockers and calcium channel blockers)
↓
HEART

LUNG
|
ANGIOTENSIN CONVERTING ENZYME (ACE)
↓

LIVER ⟶ angiotensinogen ⟶ angiostensin I
KIDNEY ⟶ renin ↑
↓
(ACE inhibitors)
↓
angiostensin II
↓
(angiostensin receptor blockers – ARBs)
↙ ↘
ADRENAL GLAND   ARTERIOLES

(vasodilators and calcium channel blockers)

aldosterone
(diuretics and aldosterone antagonists, e.g. Spironolactone)

KIDNEY ←
↓
sodium and water retention

The flow chart above will also help us when we come to look at how we can manage heart failure in Chapter 13.

Chapter 7

Congenital heart disease

This group of heart conditions are present at birth, and they are among the more common congenital conditions.

> **KEY POINTS**
> - 6–8 out of every 1,000 newborn babies has a heart defect
> - Around 5,000 children are born with a heart defect every year in the UK
> - Many mild cases are not detected until adulthood.

The causes of congenital heart disease

In fact, in the majority of cases, the cause is unknown and problems seem to occur as the result of disruption to the development of the baby's heart in the mother's womb.

The average pregnancy lasts for 40 weeks and during this time the mother will put on 28 lb in weight, on average. This amounts to around 8 lb for the baby and 20 lb for the placenta, extra fluid and any basic weight gain during the pregnancy.

In the first 20 weeks of pregnancy the baby's organs are still developing. In the second 20 weeks the baby grows. Thus, anything that interferes with the pregnancy in the early stages is liable to cause disturbance in the baby's development. If that interference is at a time when the heart is developing, then it may result in a congenital heart defect.

We tend to divide the pregnancy into three trimesters:

- First trimester (weeks 1–12)
- Second trimester (weeks 13–27)
- Third trimester (weeks 28–term).

Although a cause is not detectable in most cases, the following things can increase the risk of a baby being born with a congenital heart defect.

Genetic problems

There are several conditions that can be inherited from either or both parents, the two main ones being:

- *Down's syndrome* – this is a condition that was first described by Dr John L. H. Down, an English physician, in 1866. Babies born with it tend to have reduced muscle tone, characteristic upward slanting of the eyes, a single skin crease on their palms and be small for size at birth. There may be associated learning difficulty. It affects about 750 babies in the UK every year. Half of the children born with Down's syndrome will have a heart defect, the vast majority of which will be a septal defect (a hole in the septum – the wall between the right and left chambers of the heart – is basically what people mean when they say a 'hole in the heart'). The problem is usually caused by an extra chromosome 21 in the baby's cells – this is called 'trisomy 21' and accounts for over 90 per cent of cases of Down's syndrome. Why it occurs is not known.

- *Turner syndrome* – this is a genetic condition that causes physical abnormalities in female babies. It is caused by an abnormal sex chromosome and affects one in every 2,000 babies. About 25 per cent of those children will have a congenital heart condition.

Infections during pregnancy

Infections like colds are unlikely to do any harm to a developing baby, but influenza, if contracted in the first trimester, is associated with a doubled increase in the risk of having a baby with congenital heart disease. For this reason the flu vaccine is recommended for all pregnant women.

Rubella (German measles) is a highly infectious viral illness. Its effects on adults and children are usually quite trivial, but if it is caught by a pregnant woman that has not been immunised against it, then it can have devastating effects on the baby she is carrying. The critical time is in the first trimester. Rubella can cause multiple congenital abnormalities, including heart defects.

Other infections like Coxsackie, herpes simplex and cytomegalovirus may all cause congenital heart disease, if the mother is infected at that critical time of heart development during the first trimester.

Diabetes mellitus

Mothers with diabetes are five times more likely to have babies with congenital heart disease than are women without the condition. There are three types of diabetes:

- *Type 1 diabetes* – this used to be called 'juvenile diabetes', because it tended to occur acutely in childhood or adolescence. This is an autoimmune condition in which the immune system attacks the insulin-producing cells in the pancreas. There is therefore a deficiency of insulin and the individual will have to take insulin injections for the rest of their life. It accounts for 10 per cent of the cases of diabetes.

- *Type 2 diabetes* – where the body does not produce enough insulin, or the cells of the body fail to recognise and react to it. This used to be called 'maturity-onset diabetes', and it accounts for about 90 per cent of diabetes cases. It necessitates control either through diet, or through diet and oral medication with various hypoglycaemic (blood-sugar-lowering) drugs.

- *Gestational diabetes* – this is diabetes that starts during pregnancy, and which goes away after pregnancy finishes. It is usually discovered in the middle trimester. Since the baby has already developed its heart and organs, this form of diabetes doesn't tend to carry the same risks as types 1 and 2.

Alcohol

Drinking too much alcohol in pregnancy can cause foetal alcohol syndrome. Of those babies who develop it, about 50 per cent will have congenital heart disease. It is best avoiding alcohol during pregnancy or restricting it to about four units per week.

Iatrogenic

This means problems resulting from medication. The term comes from the Greek *iatros*, meaning 'doctor,' and *gen*, meaning 'made by'. They are problems caused by prescribed drugs taken for other conditions. The following have potential to cause congenital heart disease:

- Lithium – used to stabilise mood.
- Benzodiazepines – sedative and tranquillising drugs.
- Non-steroidal anti-inflammatory analgesics (NSAIAs) – taken to reduce inflammation.
- Acne drugs – such as isotretinoin.

The symptoms of congenital heart disease

These depend upon the condition and its severity. They also depend upon the age of the child, since the heart may become more compromised as a pump as the child gets bigger and the heart has to do more to maintain the circulation.

The problem may not be apparent immediately after birth, although if the condition is severe, it will become apparent soon after. Mild cases may go undiagnosed and not produce symptoms until teenage years.

The symptoms and signs include:

- shortness of breath
- poor feeding
- rapid heart rate
- murmur heard on listening to heart
- blueness of the lips and of the skin, which is called *cyanosis*
- finger clubbing – thickening of the ends of the fingers, like tiny clubs.

Acyanotic and cyanotic congenital heart disease

Cyanosis is the name given to a deficit in oxygen being supplied to the tissues, so that they appear blue or purple. You can see this in the skin, the mucous membranes, the lips and the fingers and toes. Congenital heart disease is often divided into two types:

- Acyanotic – in which blood from the left side of the heart, which is oxygen-rich, is mixed with deoxygenated blood from the right and then to the lungs. No discolouration occurs.
- Cyanotic – in which deoxygenated blood from the right side of the heart mixes with blood from the left side and is pumped round the body. Not enough oxygen gets to the tissues and the blue or purple appearance of the lips, skin, fingers and toes results.

ACYANOTIC CONGENITAL HEART CONDITIONS

- Persistent (or patent) ductus arteriosis
- Atrial septal defect
- Ventricular septal defect
- Pulmonary stenosis
- Coarctation of the aorta.

CYANOTIC CONGENITAL HEART CONDITIONS

- Transposition of the great vessels
- Fallot's tetralogy.

Acyanotic conditions

Persistent ductus arteriosus (PDA)

This is a condition affecting five in 100,000 newborn babies. It is due to a failure of the blood vessel that links the aorta and the pulmonary artery to close (this blood vessel is only necessary inside the womb, since the lungs of the baby have to be bypassed until birth).

The blood vessel can be closed after birth by medication. The NSAIA drugs Indomethacin or ibuprofen (a special type) can cause the ductus to close. If this fails then it can be closed by inserting a plug or coil into it via a special catheterisation.

Occasionally a PDA does not become apparent until adulthood, usually then discovered as a murmur on examination. It can still be dealt with at that stage by catheterisation and insertion of a coil or plug.

Septal defects

These are conditions in which a hole that should close by the time of birth remains between the chambers of the heart. There are two types:

- *Atrial septal defect* – in which a hole remains between the two atria. This affects 200 in every 100,000 newborn babies, or 5–10 per cent of all children born with congenital heart disease. The effect is for blood to flow into the right atrium from the left, causing the right atrium to enlarge.

- *Ventricular septal defect* – in which a hole remains between the two ventricles. This also affects 200 in every 100,000 newborn babies, or 5–10 per cent of all children born with congenital heart disease. The effect will be for blood to flow from the left to the right ventricle, causing an increase in pressure in the lungs.

Small defects may close spontaneously, but larger ones may require surgical closure.

Pulmonary stenosis

This is where the pulmonary valve, which controls the flow of blood from the right ventricle to the lungs, is narrowed, causing the right ventricle to have to work extra hard to get blood to the lungs. It affects 5–10 per cent of all children born with congenital heart disease.

Coarctation of the aorta

This is where the aorta is narrowed as it leaves the heart. The heart has to beat more forcibly to pump blood out to the tissues of the body. It may be associated with other heart defects and it affects 6–8 per cent of all children born with congenital heart disease.

It is a cause of secondary hypertension and if found in adulthood the treatment will be medical. If it is found in childhood, surgery to restore normal blood flow is likely to be advised.

Cyanotic conditions

These are more serious conditions and surgery is likely to be needed.

Transposition of the great vessels

This is a problem that arises when the pulmonary artery and the aorta are connected to the wrong chambers. Thus deoxygenated blood is pumped out to the tissues. It accounts for about 5 per cent of all children born with congenital heart disease.

The treatment required is surgery to move the vessels to the correct chambers. It is important while surgery is being prepared to keep the ductus arteriosus open in order to allow for mixing of oxygenated and deoxygenated blood. An injection of prostaglandin will help to do this.

Fallot's tetralogy

This is a serious condition in which there are four defects all at once. These are:

- a ventricular septal defect (VSD)
- pulmonary stenosis

- right ventricular hypertrophy (thickening of the right ventricle muscle)
- displaced aorta.

This affects about 30 in every 100,000 babies, and surgery is needed soon after birth in severe cases, or otherwise at about three months of age. The VSD is closed and the pulmonary valve is opened up to allow the circulation of blood to the lungs.

Chapter 8

Valvular heart disease

The heart valves develop in a baby between the fourth and seventh weeks of pregancy, so any of the adverse factors we looked at in the last chapter on congenital heart disease could potentially affect the development of the valves.

The four heart valves

The valves between the chambers of the heart are not identical. For one thing, they have different numbers of cusps (the flaps that open and shut). When those cusps open they allow flow of blood either from one atrium to its corresponding ventricle, or from the left ventricle to the rest of the body, or the right ventricle to the lungs. They only allow flow in one direction and when they are closed, they should not allow any leakage.

The valves are:

- *Tricuspid valve* – a valve with three cusps that allows blood to flow from the right atrium into the right ventricle.

- *Pulmonary valve* – a valve with three cusps that allows blood to flow from the right ventricle to the lungs through the pulmonary artery.
- *Mitral valve* – a two-cusp valve that allows blood to flow from the left atrium into the left ventricle.
- *Aortic valve* – a three-cusp valve that allows blood to flow from the left ventricle into the aorta and then to the rest of the body.

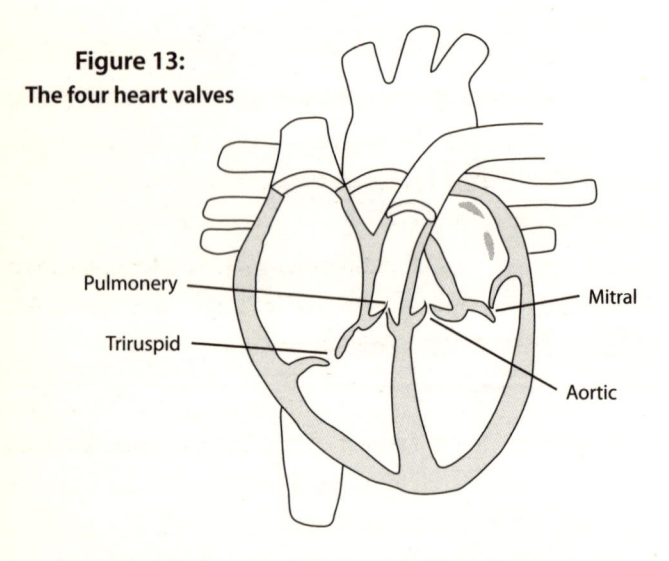

Figure 13:
The four heart valves

Pulmonery

Triruspid

Mitral

Aortic

The tricuspid and the mitral are referred to as atrioventricular (AV) valves, because they allow blood to flow from the atria to the ventricles, but not in the other direction.

The pulmonary and aortic are called semilunar valves, because they are shaped like half-moons. They allow blood to flow out of the heart from the ventricles to the two exiting arteries, the pulmonary artery and the aorta, but not in the other direction.

Figure 14: The valves in cross-section to show the directions they open

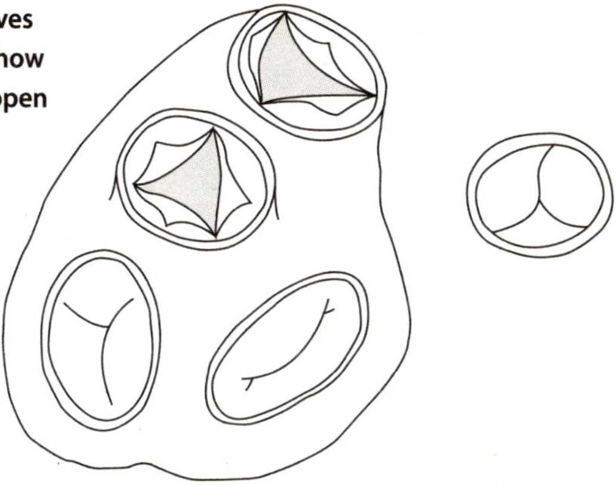

Two main problems can occur with a valve:

- *Stenosis* – when the valve becomes narrowed and blood cannot easily flow into the next chamber or into the blood vessel. The heart has to pump harder to get blood through.

- *Incompetence* – when the valve leaks, so that blood flows backwards, throwing pressure on the chamber that is on the receiving end.

The causes of valvular heart disease

There are several main causes:

- *Congenital* – especially pulmonary stenosis and aortic stenosis.
- *Rheumatic* – as a result of scarring caused by rheumatic fever or rheumatic heart disease. This is a condition that occurs about

six weeks after a streptococcal infection. It is relatively rare these days because of antibiotic prescribing. It is possible that it might increase in the years to come, however, since antibiotic prescribing is being reduced in response to the increasing problem of antibiotic resistance. This condition mainly affects the mitral and aortic valves.

- *Ageing and calcification* – this mainly affects the aortic valve in the elderly to produce aortic stenosis.

- *Cardiomyopathy* – this is disease of the heart muscle. It may have been something that the person was born with or it may have been acquired from rheumatic heart disease or subacute bacterial endocarditis. It can affect the valves by causing swelling of the heart muscle to obstruct flow through a particular valve, or it can cause dilation of the heart and stretching of valve rings to make the valves leak or become incompetent.

- *Subacute bacterial endocarditis* – this is an infection of the lining of the heart that can complicate any of the above conditions and causes further scarring of the valves.

- *Syphilis* – this used to be a main cause of valvular heart disease, but it is less common in western society. It is still common throughout the world and must still be considered a potential cause.

The symptoms of valvular heart disease

These are variable, depending on the severity of the valve problem.

Mitral valve disease

Both mitral stenosis and mitral incompetence are commoner in women:

Mitral stenosis

This can produce the following symptoms:

- Fatigue
- Breathlessness on exertion
- Frequent bronchitis in the winter
- Right-sided heart failure
- Palpitations or irregular heart rhythm, especially atrial fibrillation.

Atrial fibrillation puts the person at a very real risk of having a stroke. There is also significant risk of heart failure.

Mitral incompetence

This is often called mitral regurgitation. The problem here is that blood leaks backwards and the left side of the heart can become overloaded to produce left-sided heart failure. Atrial fibrillation can also occur with mitral incompetence.

Aortic valve disease

Both aortic stenosis and aortic incompetence can occur. Aortic valve disease is most common in middle-aged men:

Aortic stenosis

This tends to reduce the cardiac output, since it is harder to pump blood out of the heart through the narrowed valve. It can produce the following symptoms:

- Weakness and fainting
- Angina

Aortic incompetence

These patients may have no symptoms for many years, but then develop breathlessness on exertion or even breathlessness lying flat (orthopnoea). This is because they have developed left-sided heart failure.

Endocarditis – the problem that valvular heart disease can cause

Damaged heart valves can be sites in which infections such as endocarditis can develop. Endocarditis is an inflammation of the endocardium, the lining of the heart that covers the whole of the chambers and the valves themselves.

It can be caused by streptococcal or staphylococcal bacteria. Streptococcus viridans is one such organism that lives in the mouth and can enter the bloodstream during dental procedures.

Endocarditis can occur suddenly, when it is called acute bacterial endocarditis. If it occurs gradually, over weeks and months, it is called subacute bacterial endocarditis. Either way, it can cause further damage to the heart and is a serious condition that needs treatment, since it can be life threatening in 10–25 per cent of cases.

> Bacteria can enter the bloodstream from all sorts of infections, so if you have a heart-valve problem and are about to undergo a procedure, especially dentistry, it may be advisable for you to have an antibiotic beforehand.
>
> **In fact, if you have a valvular problem, you should always alert doctors or dentists to that fact before having any procedure.**

Assessment

The different valvular conditions can be picked up by a GP when listening to the heart, because they all produce characteristic heart murmurs. It is beyond the scope of this book to go into the differences between them, but the important thing is to identify the presence of a murmur and then have it investigated fully, probably by a cardiologist.

The following investigations can all be useful:

- *ECG* – an electrocardiogram to show the electrical activity of the heart and to assess the rhythm of the heart.

- *Chest X-ray* – to show the shape and size of the heart and to exclude other problems.

- *Echocardiogram (or just 'echo')* – a test using sound waves to build up a picture of the heart as it beats. It shows the heart pumping and also shows the functioning of the valves.

- *Transoesophageal echocardiogram* – this is a special type of echocardiogram in which an ultrasound transducer is passed down the oesophagus to get an even clearer view of the heart.

- *CT scan or MRI scan* – these can both give a very good picture of the heart and the valves.

- *Angiogram* – a catheter is inserted into the heart via an artery and dye is injected. This gives a clearer X-ray view of the heart valves.

Treatment of valvular heart disease

There may not be any need for treatment, but most cases will be treated either by drugs or by heart surgery, or sometimes with a combination of surgery and drugs. The drugs that may be needed include:

- *Antihypertensives* – to treat high blood pressure.
- *Diuretics* – to remove fluid and alleviate heart failure.
- *ACE inhibitors* – which are antihypertensive and also help in the treatment of heart failure.
- *Digoxin* – to help with the regulation of heart rhythm.

- *Anticoagulants* – such as warfarin, which helps reduce the risk of blood clots forming.

Heart surgery

There are a number of procedures that may be undertaken, including the following:

- *Valve repair or replacement* – surgery may involve the replacement of a valve with an artificial one, and sometimes surgery may be suggested to repair a valve. Valve repair may be preferable to valve replacement, since there is less likelihood of infection and the strength and power of the heart will not be impaired.
- *Balloon valvuloplasty* – used to enlarge a stenosed (narrowed) valve, it involves a catheter being introduced into the heart via a blood vessel. It is then manoeuvred into the relevant valve and a small balloon is inflated to widen that valve. This procedure is only normally used for children or young adults.

Chapter 9

Other diseases of the heart

There are several other conditions that either affect the heart directly or which affect the heart as part of a multi-system condition.

Cardiomyopathy

This term means disease of the heart muscle, from the Greek *kardia*, meaning 'heart', *myo*, meaning 'muscle', and *pathos*, meaning 'disease'.

It is a condition that can be common within families, or which seems to affect some members of the family but not others. It can affect people of any age and most often it is an inherited condition.

It is not possible at this time to cure cardiomyopathy, but it is treatable and one can lead a full and long life with it.

Types of cardiomyopathy

There are several types of inherited cardiomyopathy affecting people throughout the world, but in the West, there are three main types.

Hypertrophic cardiomyopathy (HCM)

This is a condition that causes thickening of the heart muscle, hypertrophy being a process where the individual muscle fibres become enlarged. It is often referred to as HCM or HOCUM, and it is a genetic condition that affects about two in every thousand people in the UK population, although not all will have symptoms. It will affect around half of the children of people who have HCM.

It may cause the following symptoms:

- Shortness of breath
- Chest pain
- Palpitations
- Faintness

It can also cause heart failure, as some patients with HCM may develop problems with the mitral valve and develop arrhythmias.

Treatment is possible with the drugs that are available to treat hypertension or abnormal rhythms. If there are significant problems with heart rhythm, then a pacemaker may be needed.

In very severe cases, if there is a risk of cardiac arrest, then a device called an implantable cardioverter defibrillator (ICD) can be inserted under the collarbone. It is a small device the size of a matchbox and it detects abnormalities in rhythm and will pace the heart, or even defibrillate it to restart a normal rhythm.

Dilated cardiomyopathy (DCM)

This is a disease of the heart muscle where the heart muscle does not get thicker, but instead gets thinner and stretched. The heart cannot, as a result, pump the circulation effectively.

This can be an inherited condition, which affects around one half of the children of people who have DCM. It can also develop secondary to:

- Alcohol excess
- Viral infections such as Coxsackie B
- Uncontrolled hypertension
- Cardiotoxic drugs
- Connective tissue diseases, e.g. systemic lupus erythematosus
- Endocrine (hormone-secreting gland) disorders, such as hypothyroidism, hyperthyroidism and acromegaly
- Muscular dystrophy
- Pregnancy.

DCM can cause heart failure and therefore present with shortness of breath, swelling of the ankles and abdomen, tiredness, fatigue, palpitations and irregular heart rhythms.

As with HCM, treatment is possible with the drugs that are available to treat hypertension or abnormal rhythms. If there are significant problems with heart rhythm, then a pacemaker may be needed.

In very severe cases, again as with HCM, if there is a risk of cardiac arrest then a device called an implantable cardioverter defibrillator (ICD) can be inserted under the collarbone. It is a small device the size of a matchbox and it detects abnormalities in rhythm and will pace the heart, or even defibrillate it to restart a normal rhythm.

Arrhythmogenic right ventricular cardiomyopathy (ARVC)

This is a rare inherited condition affecting the heart muscle. Some people have no symptoms from it, but others have major problems. It tends to affect the right ventricle, which gets thin and inefficient, so the heart does not pump blood adequately to the lungs. It may also cause abnormal rhythms of the heart.

Sometimes the condition does not become apparent until later in life, when it presents as abnormal heart rhythms or heart failure.

All three of the cardiomyopathies are treatable, but they do need supervision by a cardiologist.

Myocarditis

This is an inflammation of the myocardium. It may be the result of an infection with a virus, such as Coxsackie. It can also be caused by diphtheria, rheumatic fever or use of drugs such as cocaine.

The presentation is usually acute, with chest pain, and it may even mimic a myocardial infarction. It can also cause heart failure or even sudden death. Many people make a complete recovery, but others may need long-term treatment to control heart failure or abnormal heart rhythms.

Pericarditis

This is an inflammation of the sac that envelops the heart (the function of the sac is to anchor the heart in one place and stop it moving freely about the chest – it has two layers separated by a thin film of fluid that lubricates them both).

Pericarditis is caused by:

- *Viral infection* – the majority of cases are viral, e.g. Coxsackie virus, echoviruses (which are found in the gastrointestinal tract), mumps virus, influenza viruses, hepatitis virus and HIV.

- *Bacterial infection* – this will produce pus between the layers of the sac and the sac can go stiff as a result. This then inhibits the movement of the heart.

- *Tuberculosis (TB)* – this can cause pericarditis, but usually only when the condition is quite advanced and has significantly affected the lungs.

- *Post-myocardial infarction* – this is one of the potential complications of a heart attack.

- *Kidney failure* – pericarditis can occur as a complication of kidney failure when waste products build up.

- *Trauma* – such as a stab wound to the chest.

- *Cancer* – either cancer of the lung or a distant spread from another cancer.

- *Radiotherapy* – for any cancer of the chest.

- *Inflammatory conditions* – such as rheumatoid arthritis, polyarteritis nodosa (swollen or damaged arteries), scleroderma (an autoimmune skin disease) or systemic lupus erythematosus (connective tissue disease).

The main symptoms of pericarditis are chest pain and a fever. The chest pain can be sharp and incapacitating and may mimic a myocardial infarction. The pain may be worse on deep inspiration or on swallowing or coughing, and it should be dealt with as an emergency to exclude other conditions.

Complications of pericarditis

The majority of cases resolve spontaneously within a few weeks and can be treated with simple anti-inflammatory drugs, but some cases may lead to more serious conditions:

- *Cardiac effusion* – in some cases the fluid accumulation between the two layers of the sac can be so extensive that it can impede the pumping of the heart.

- *Cardiac tamponade* – this is a potentially life-threatening condition when the cardiac effusion is so extensive that it inhibits the beating of the heart. The cardiac effusion must be released by being drained.

- *Constrictive pericarditis* – if for some reason the inflammation lasts for a long time, then the pericardium can become thickened and inelastic, and it even may need to be removed surgically.

PART TWO

DEALING WITH HEART DISEASE

You can look after your heart

We often take our health for granted. Many people adopt a fatalistic view of life and think that what will be, will be. That may cause them to ignore the risk of developing angina or having a heart attack. Yet the simple fact is that many heart attacks are avoidable, and that means that a lot of early deaths from heart attacks could also be avoided.

As we shall see in this part of the book, there are lots of things that one can do to reduce the risk of developing a heart problem. Similarly, there are lots of things that can be done once angina has developed, or after one has suffered from a heart attack.

Chapter 10

Understanding your risk of having a heart attack

In assessing the likelihood of anyone having a heart attack or of developing angina, we look at their risk factors. It is important to appreciate that by adopting a healthy lifestyle you can reduce your risk of having a coronary event.

> **SOME NATIONAL COMPARISONS**
>
> There is enormous variation in the incidence of heart disease in different countries, as can be seen from the following death rates: [11]
>
> - Slovakia   216 per 100,000 people
> - UK   112 per 100,000 people
> - USA   106 per 100,000 people
> - France   39 per 100,000 people
> - Japan   30 per 100,000 people

From the figures in the above box you can see that some countries have very low incidences. France has always been a bit of a conundrum, since the French diet would seem to have a high fat content, yet the death rate from heart disease is very low. This is known as the 'French paradox'. One theory is that it may relate to their use of wine with meals.

Risk factors for coronary heart disease

As we shall see, there are several risk factors for coronary heart disease. In assessing overall risk, it is important to realise that it is not just one risk factor that is assessed, but the total picture provided by all of them together. If someone has a very healthy lifestyle and scores high on one risk factor alone, then it may be decided not to treat them. Some of the following risk factors cannot be altered, yet many others can. First of all, let us look at those factors that you cannot control.

Non-modifiable risk factors

Genetic make-up

Some families seem to have more members suffering from angina or have more heart attacks than others. There may be something in their genes that predisposes certain people to those conditions. Having said that, there are no readily available tests that can conclusively predict whether one will have a heart attack.

Some people have a genetic predisposition to a raised cholesterol level. We call this familial hypercholesterolaemia. We can't change the genes, but we can reduce the cholesterol, and we shall return to this in the section that covers modifiable risk factors.

There is also a genetic condition called homocystinuria, in which raised levels of an amino acid occur. This tends to promote endothelial damage to the lining of blood vessels and as a result predisposes the person to atherosclerosis.

The simple fact is that if you do have a family that has a higher incidence of heart problems, then you should see your doctor to have your overall risk rated, and then you should try to reduce your risk from the factors that you can do something about.

Gender and age

Males generally have a higher risk than females and they tend to manifest it earlier. However, in middle age there is a slight increased risk for women over men. It seems that this relates to hormonal change around the menopause, and possibly to the fact that women may be taking hormone replacement therapy (HRT) during the menopause (female hormones seem to have a protective effect against coronary heart disease but after the menopause, when female hormone levels fall, that protective effect is lost). By the age of 65, the risk is about equal for both sexes.

KEY POINTS

A family history is considered to be most relevant if:

- a first-degree male relative has angina or has a heart attack before the age of 55
- a first-degree female relative has angina or has a heart attack before the age of 65.

Ethnic background

Coronary heart disease occurs in all ethnic backgrounds, but people of African, African-Caribbean or South Asian origin are at increased risk. Why this is the case is unclear, but it may relate to higher levels of blood pressure, dietary factors or inherited tendencies.

> **ETHRISK**
>
> The ETHRISK is a test tool that can be used to calculate the risk of heart disease and stroke in British black and minority ethnic groups. It is used for people aged 35 to 74 without diabetes or a past history of cerebrovascular disease. It is based on sex, age, systolic blood pressure, cholesterol levels and smoking status. Your general practitioner will be able to discuss this, if requested.

Modifiable risk factors

These are the risks that you **can** control.

Smoking

The smoking habit has no health benefits whatsoever, but greatly increases the risk of developing many potentially lethal conditions, including heart attack and stroke.

> **KEY POINTS**
> - Smoking increases the risk of coronary heart disease by 50 per cent.

- Moderate smokers have a 60 per cent greater chance of dying from cardiovascular disease than non-smokers.
- Heavy smokers (more than 20 cigarettes a day) have an 85 per cent greater chance of dying from cardiovascular disease than non-smokers.[12]
- Smokers have double the risk of having a stroke as non-smokers have.
- Tobacco-smoking is the single biggest cause of lung cancer (about 90–95 per cent of cases).
- People who smoke 20 or more cigarettes a day are 20 times more likely to develop lung cancer than non-smokers.
- Only 25 per cent of people diagnosed with lung cancer will survive longer than a year.
- Passive smoking increases the risk of coronary heart disease by 25 per cent.
- The benefits of stopping smoking begin instantly! It seems that the greatest benefit will accrue, the younger you are when you stop.

Hypertension

Uncontrolled high blood pressure (or hypertension) is the biggest risk factor for stroke. It is sensible for all adults to have their blood pressure recorded at least once every five years, since high blood pressure is an insidious condition that can creep up on an individual without them having any symptoms whatsoever. If your blood pressure is borderline, then your doctor will recommend having it checked more frequently.

As we saw in Chapter 4, hypertension affects about a billion people worldwide and in the UK the prevalence of hypertension has been estimated to be 42 per cent in the population aged 35 to 64. Preventing high blood pressure is well worthwhile to reduce one's future risk of heart attack or stroke.

Cholesterol

Most people know that a high cholesterol level in the blood is not good for you. It can increase the risk of heart disease or of having a stroke. It is not just the level of cholesterol that matters, however, but the relative balance between good cholesterol and bad cholesterol. Essentially, the lower the level of bad cholesterol the lower your risk.

Cholesterol is a type of waxy, fat substance that is found in all of the cells of the body. It is in fact an important substance for the body, but you just don't want too much of it. Cholesterol is carried around the bloodstream in packets called lipoproteins – the lipo is the inside part of the package and consists of fat; the protein is the outer part. There are two types of lipoprotein which carry your cholesterol; low-density lipoprotein (LDL), commonly known as the bad cholesterol; and high-density lipoprotein (HDL), commonly thought of as good cholesterol.

The problem with too much LDL cholesterol (bad cholesterol) is that it tends to cause a build-up of cholesterol in your artery walls. Imagine that the lining of an artery is like a sponge with lots of small holes in it. Think of the LDL cholesterol as a small ball, about the size of the holes in the sponge. By contrast, HDL cholesterol is like a much bigger ball, much larger than the holes. So, if you have blood carrying a mixture of both types of ball, a large proportion of the small balls will lodge in the holes. The larger ones will just bounce off and carry on their way. That is how bad cholesterol attaches itself to your blood vessels.

Recent research from the USA has shown that when people eat cholesterol-lowering foods in addition to going on a low-fat diet they can reduce the bad cholesterol by 13 per cent, as opposed to a mere 3 per cent when they only reduce the fat content. The beneficial foods are: those containing plant sterols, such as nuts; foods with viscous fibre, such as barley and oats; the soy protein found in soya milk, tofu and soy meat substitutes; oily fish (such as salmon, trout, herrings and sardines); fresh fruit and vegetables; and pulses.

If your cholesterol level is found to be high, you should do all that you can to reduce it. There are various dietary things that may help, as can exercise, but for many people it will require one of the statin group of drugs, which we'll consider in Chapter 11.

LIPID PROFILE

- The blood test for fats in the blood is called a lipid profile. It measures HDL cholesterol, LDL cholesterol, total cholesterol, triglycerides (another type of blood fat that needs to be maintained at a healthy level) and cholesterol to HDL ratio (see below).
- Lipids are measured in millimoles per litre (mmol/l).
- It is desirable for total cholesterol to be under 5 mmol/l.
- In the cholesterol:HDL ratio, ideally the HDL should be higher than 20 per cent of the total (i.e. 1 mmol/l or more). This can be confusing, but suppose the cholesterol level is 6 mmol/l (which is high) and the HDL is 1 mmol/l, then the ratio would be 6:1. That means that the overall cholesterol is too high and the HDL is not high enough, because most of the cholesterol is in the form of the bad cholesterol LDL. On the other hand, if the cholesterol level is 6 and the HDL is 3, then the ratio is 6:3, which is 2:1. This means that there is a good proportion of the HDL, which is good.

Obesity

It is known that increasing levels of obesity are associated with increased incidence of heart disease. It seems likely that just being obese increases the individual's risk, yet it is not known whether it is the obesity itself or other factors that cause the increase. The sort of secondary risk factors that might come into play are diabetes, raised cholesterol and possibly hypertension. Nonetheless, as a marker of general health, it is as well to try to keep your weight to a healthy level.

Ideally you should aim for a Body Mass Index (BMI) of 25. BMI is an accepted means of relating weight to height. It is worked out by dividing your weight in kg by the square of your height in metres. You can find BMI calculators on the Internet. It is essentially giving an estimation of human body fat, although it does not actually measure fat.

The early-death rate of people who are 14–18 kg (30–40 lb) overweight is 30 per cent greater than one would expect in a general population of people of normal weight. More alarmingly, there is a 50 per cent increase in early death for men who weigh more than 40 per cent above ideal body weight.

IT IS BETTER TO BE A PEAR THAN AN APPLE

You may have heard this one. It relates to the distribution of your excess body fat. Fat accumulated around the abdomen, the classic 'beer belly', has a high correlation with the risk of coronary heart disease.

This can be measured by comparing the ratio of the waist with the hips. A high waist-to-hips ratio (beer belly) will tend to make one look like an apple. By contrast, a slimmer abdomen and larger hips has a lower waist-to-hips ratio and a lower risk.

It really is better to be a pear than an apple.

A measurement of obesity that is perhaps more accurate than BMI (which isn't all that easy to calculate) is the waist-to-height ratio. That is your waist measurement over your height. It should be less than 0.5 to give a low risk. Once it gets above this 0.5 ratio then the individual has too much central body fat and is overweight. This is associated with an increased risk, and the greater the figure the greater the risk. It seems to be a better indicator, because the BMI makes no distinction between muscle and fat. The waist-to-height ratio, on the other hand, is purely an indicator of your body proportions.

This was demonstrated by researchers at Oxford Brookes University[13], who examined data on patients whose BMI and waist-to-height ratio were measured in the 1980s. Twenty years later, death rates among the group were much more closely linked to participants' earlier waist-to-height ratio than their BMI, suggesting it is a more useful tool for identifying health risks at an early stage.

> **KEY POINT**
>
> As a rule of thumb, a waist circumference of more than 40 inches for men and 35 inches for women indicates a high risk of coronary heart disease.

Inactivity and lack of exercise

This is really just common sense. The less active a person is, the less fit they are likely to be. They are then more likely to put on weight and to lose the tone in their muscles. It becomes a vicious circle.

The benefits of regular exercise are well known in terms of helping to reduce the risk of various ailments, including heart disease and stroke. For one thing it helps to control weight, and it also helps to reduce cholesterol and the risk of developing diabetes.

In terms of losing weight, people often think that its value is simply a matter of burning calories. It is not as simple as that. Exercise has quite a profound effect on the body by virtue of what it does to the metabolism – it seems to stimulate a hormone called 'irisin', named after Iris, the Greek messenger goddess, because it seems to deliver a message from the muscles that stimulates amazing changes in the body.

Scientists found this hormone in the membranes of muscle cells when they were investigating a particular gene, and they were aware that exercise somehow switched this gene on. Having found the hormone, they used lab cultures and mice to show that irisin has a powerful effect on white adipose tissue, the type of fat that accumulates under the skin and contributes to obesity. The irisin causes the body to convert white fat to brown fat, and brown fat is regarded as 'good' fat, because it burns off more calories than exercise alone.

In the mice studies, the researchers found that not only was white fat converted into brown fat, but also that irisin had a positive effect on glucose tolerance. This could be of vital importance as a treatment in the future, since the link between obesity and diabetes is well known.

In practical terms it is worth incorporating exercise into your day. This does not have to mean going to a gym. You can do it simply by walking more. A study from Missouri looked at the effect of short bursts of exercise on a group of men and women who did not regularly exercise. Over the trial period, on three occasions, they were given a high-fat meal, consisting of a milkshake with heavy whipping cream. Before one of the meals they exercised vigorously for 30 consecutive minutes. Another time they exercised for three ten-minute sessions with breaks in between. On the last occasion, they did not exercise. Interestingly, the short bursts of activity, equivalent to three brisk ten-minute walks, had the best effect in lowering the blood-fat levels.

Diet

We shall look at this in more detail in Chapter 18, but here is a quick summary of the main points to keep you going in the meantime:

> **KEY POINTS**
> - Fat consumption should be less than 30 per cent of the total calorific intake.
> - Junk food rich in trans fats should be kept to a minimum.
> - Salt intake should be restricted to a safe level.
> - Oily fish should ideally be eaten three times a week.
> - Five fruit or vegetable portions should be eaten every day.

Alcohol and the J-shaped curve

A little alcohol a day seems to be beneficial in reducing the risk of coronary heart disease. Too much, on the other hand, increases the risk.

This trend can be seen in the J-shaped curve phenomenon in Figure 15, which shows the risk of death from coronary heart disease when measured against an average number of alcoholic drinks a day. At the start, with people who have drunk no alcohol, their death risk is standard. Then, with moderate drinking, the risk drops, then it increases as the average number of daily drinks increases.

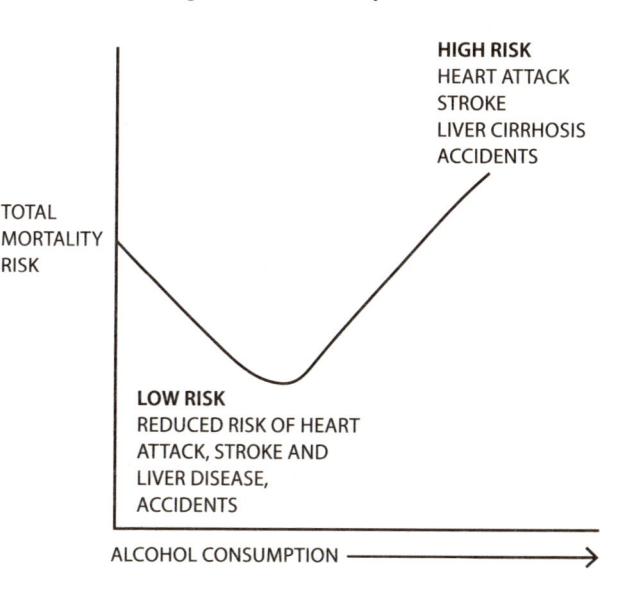

Figure 15: The J-shaped alcohol curve

TOTAL MORTALITY RISK

HIGH RISK
HEART ATTACK
STROKE
LIVER CIRRHOSIS
ACCIDENTS

LOW RISK
REDUCED RISK OF HEART ATTACK, STROKE AND LIVER DISEASE, ACCIDENTS

ALCOHOL CONSUMPTION ⟶

KEY POINTS

The Royal College of Physicians recommends that:

- Men should not drink more than 21 units of alcohol a week and their daily alcohol intake should not exceed three to four units.
- Women should not drink more than 14 units a week and their daily alcohol intake should not exceed two to three units.
- Continued drinking at the upper limit is not advised, and at least two alcohol-free days a week should be taken.
- As a rule of thumb, heavy drinking is defined as six units in six hours.
- A unit is either a small measure of spirit, a small glass of wine or a half pint of beer or lager.

Stress and negative emotions

Stress and negative emotions can both have an effect on a person and do seem to increase the risk of heart disease. It is impossible to quantify this, yet research does show that some negative emotions, like anger, can have a direct effect on the heart. We shall look at this in more depth when we come to consider the life cycle in Chapter 17.

Inflammation

Much research work is being done on the relationship between the chronic inflammation that is a feature of other conditions (like arthritis or inflammatory bowel conditions) and heart disease. Logically, inflammation is associated with increased risk, since inflammation is one of the factors that predisposes to and even causes atherosclerosis.

Research is ongoing to determine whether conditions like rheumatoid arthritis, psoriasis and chronic gum disease could be associated with increased risk and, if so, what can be done about that.

Diabetes mellitus

Diabetes is a disorder of metabolism in which a person has a high blood-sugar count. This can be either because insulin production by the pancreas is inadequate, or because the body cells do not properly respond to it. The main symptoms of diabetes are increased thirst and a frequent desire to pass urine.

The condition was known to the Ancient Egyptians and the Ancient Greeks. Indeed, the second-century Greek physician Aretaeus introduced the term 'diabetes', meaning 'syphon', because of the fact that people drank lots of water and seemed to siphon it through their system.

Dr Thomas Willis, the physician to King Charles II, discovered that the urine of diabetic people tasted sweet. It was he who added the second name, 'mellitus', from the Latin for honey.

> **KEY POINT**
> - Diabetes at least doubles the risk of having a heart attack.

Cold weather

It has been recognised for several decades that mortality rises by 19 per cent between the months of December and March in the UK. The majority of these deaths are due to cardiac deaths and strokes and respiratory problems, rather than hypothermia.

In 1984 Professor W. R. Keatinge demonstrated in the laboratory that cold environments caused definite changes in the blood and blood pressure.14 He showed that there is an increase in platelet and red blood cell counts and an increase in blood viscosity. The blood pressure also begins to rise. Since all of these factors can increase the risk of having a heart attack or a stroke, especially in the elderly and in those with underlying circulatory problems, a Cold Weather Plan is in operation in England.

The Cold Weather Plan is a public health plan for health and social care services and professionals to prepare for and prevent unnecessary deaths among those at risk during the winter months. It also aims to alert and prepare individuals to protect themselves in order to reduce their risk.

There are four Cold Weather Alerts and the Cold Weather Plan sets out the actions that should be taken at each level.

An easy-to-read pamphlet is available from the NHS on this website: www.gov.uk/government/uploads/system/uploads/attachment_data/file/216644/dh_133112.pdf. This gives good advice about the Cold Weather Plan.

Essentially, if you are at risk, then ensure that you have any preventive injections, including for flu or other infections, that you are eligible for. You can check this with your GP or practice nurse. Importantly, make sure that your home is warm with a temperature of at least 21°C (70°F) during the day and 18°C (65°F) at night. Many people may not feel cold, but if the temperature drops below these levels then changes in the blood viscosity and an increase in blood pressure may occur, without you being aware of it.

Cardiovascular risk assessment

At your GP's surgery you may be offered a cardiovascular risk assessment. This may be done by the GP, or more usually by the practice nurse. This is usually offered to people aged from 40 to 74 and involves a consultation during which information is gathered about you, looking at all of the potential risk factors that we have discussed in this chapter. This will broadly look at lifestyle including smoking history, alcohol intake, diet and family history of cardiovascular disease. A history of cardiovascular disease (a heart attack, angina, stroke or mini-stroke) that occurred in a close male relative under the age of 55 years or a close female relative of 65 years or less would be taken into account in working out your own risk.

Blood tests will be carried out to measure lipids, including cholesterol, and possibly blood sugar (if diabetes is a risk factor).

Height and weight will be recorded, as will your blood pressure.

A follow-up appointment after about a week is generally arranged to discuss the findings and to give you a risk rating, based upon which you will be allocated to one of three groups:

- *Low risk* – less than 10 per cent chance of having coronary heart disease in the next ten years.
- *Intermediate risk* – 10–20 per cent chance of having a coronary event in the next ten years.
- *High risk* – greater than 20 per pent chance of having a coronary event within ten years.

With low risk, which does not mean 'no risk', advice would be given about maintaining the risk at that level.

With moderate risk, individual risk factors that may be modifiable (such as smoking, alcohol intake, or insufficient exercise) may be looked at.

With high risk, it may be that drug treatment to control blood-cholesterol levels with statins may be suggested, or ways in which to control blood pressure may be considered. Or further investigation may be indicated, and we will look at what sort of investigations might be appropriate in the next chapter. Some may be offered in the surgery, but others will necessitate a visit to a hospital or other outpatient unit.

Chapter 11

What could this chest pain be? Is it angina?

As described in Chapter 5, there are four main ways in which coronary heart disease manifests itself. These are:

- Angina

- Heart attack, also known as a myocardial infarction (MI)

- Heart failure

- Arrhythmias (irregular beating of the heart).

It is not possible to predict which of these will occur. Although we understand that they can all have the same underlying cause, arteriosclerosis, it is not clear why one person develops angina while another goes into heart failure.

The symptoms to look out for

The following symptoms may be highly significant so if you develop them (and particularly if they are severe or persistent) you should seek medical help to get a diagnosis:

Chest pain – typically, central chest pain with radiation to the neck or down the left arm suggests cardiac pain. If it is associated with clamminess and faintness then emergency medical help should be called for, because that could be a heart attack. If the pain goes away, but is provoked by exertion and eased by rest, then that could be angina.

Palpitations – the sensation of the heart beating rapidly inside the chest may be normal. This can occur if you have had too much coffee, too many stimulants or if you are stressed. If it is continuous or feels irregular, or is associated with shortness of breath, then medical help is advisable. It is possible that it is caused by coronary artery disease depriving the conductive part of the heart of oxygen, causing it to go into an abnormal rhythm.

Shortness of breath at night, while lying flat, or on mild exertion may indicate heart failure.

Swelling of the ankles as the day goes on could also indicate heart failure.

> **KEY POINT – EMERGENCY TREATMENT**
>
> If you experience a severe chest pain and have never had one before, this is an indication of the need for emergency assessment. That means calling 999 to be admitted to hospital – don't wait, since time may be of the essence if you are having a heart attack.

Angina – a general description

This is a severe chest pain that is experienced on exertion, such as lifting or going uphill. It usually only lasts two or three minutes, but goes away on rest. It starts in the left side of the chest and radiates into the left arm or up into the neck and the throat. Chest pain is angina until proven otherwise.

In assessing your condition, doctors form a differential diagnosis, which is essentially a league table of the likely diagnoses or of all the possible causes of a clutch of symptoms. In the case of chest pains, angina is top of the list and it is the first thing to exclude or confirm.

Your GP

This is often the first person that you see, especially if you have had some chest pains that settled spontaneously and you want to check whether they were significant or not. Your GP will take a history and give you a physical examination, including taking your pulse, listening to your heart with a stethoscope and taking your blood pressure. He will be listening to check that the heart is in normal rhythm, that there are no signs of heart failure or congestion in the lungs, and that there are no heart murmurs present.

An ECG will be needed and will be done in the surgery.

The ECG

The electrocardiogram is the name of the test used to record the electrical activity of the heart. It is sometimes also referred to as an electrocardiograph, but the common abbreviation of ECG is standard. The machine is essentially a galvanometer, which records the electrical potential between two points in the heart.

The principle that it all works on is that when any muscle is stimulated there is a change in electrical potential along the muscle fibre. This is picked up by the ECG machine.

The patient is connected to the machine by wires attached to electrodes that are strapped on to the limbs. The right and left arms and the left leg are recording electrodes. The one on the right leg is used to earth the patient. Chest leads are also used and are labelled as V1 to V6 (see Figure 16).

Including those six chest leads, the standard ECG has 12 leads (or segments) in total, and a long strip to record the rhythm of the heart. This means that the recording is allowed to run over several heartbeats in order to measure the regularity of the beats.

There are three bipolar leads:

- Lead I records the difference in potential between the right and left arms.

- Lead II records the difference in potential between the right arm and left leg.

- Lead III records the difference in potential between the left arm and the left leg.

- And there are three unipolar leads, which are also referred to as 'augmented leads':

- The aVR lead from the right arm.
- The aVL lead from the left arm.
- The aVF lead from the left leg.

These three leads are called unipolar or augmented leads because they record from one limb only and, because the voltage is therefore too small to be recorded, they are boosted, or 'augmented', to produce a deflection on the ECG that can be seen and compared against each other.

The individual leads (or segments) of the ECG effectively 'look at' the heart from different directions, as in Figure 16. This allows the doctor to see which part of the heart has been affected.

Figure 16: The different ECG leads 'look' at the heart from different directions

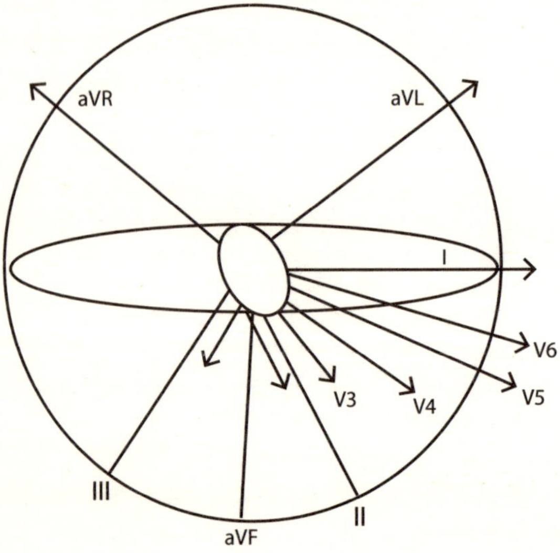

The trace of the heart will show a series of spikes, and the individual heartbeat is thus recorded. We looked at it in Chapter 1 in the section on the electrical conducting system of the heart and in Figure 2, showing the ECG tracing.

The resting ECG

- This is the ECG taken with the patient lying down. With angina, the ECG may look perfectly normal during attacks, in that it shows no signs of ischaemia.

- If the ECG is taken during an attack it may show ST depression or T wave inversion or tall peaked T waves, as in Figure 17. These are signs of ischaemia.

- If the resting ECG does not show anything untoward and the doctor still thinks that stable angina is likely, then further testing is needed. This will usually result in a referral to a rapid access chest pain clinic at the local hospital.

- If the resting ECG shows definite signs of myocardial ischaemia then an acute coronary syndrome is diagnosed and the patient should be admitted to hospital.

As we saw in Chapter 5, angina is differentiated into:

- Stable angina
- Unstable angina
- Crescendo angina
- Decubitus angina.

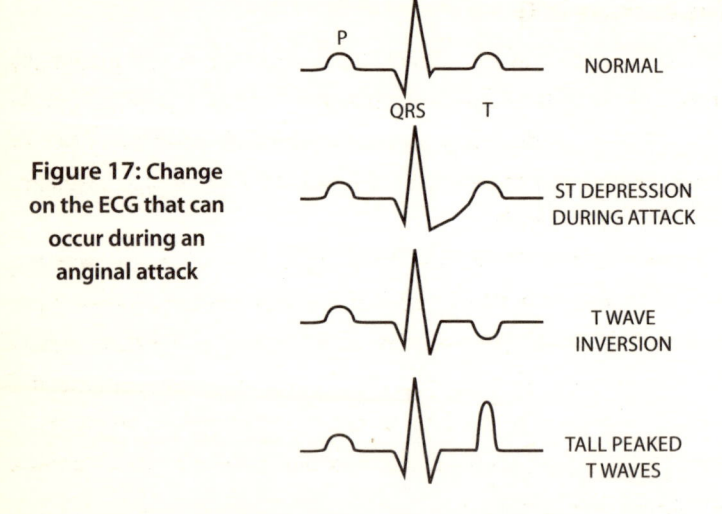

Figure 17: Change on the ECG that can occur during an anginal attack

- NORMAL (P, QRS, T)
- ST DEPRESSION DURING ATTACK
- T WAVE INVERSION
- TALL PEAKED T WAVES

If stable angina is diagnosed, then the GP may investigate and treat, or an appointment may be arranged at the rapid access chest pain clinic. If any of the other types are diagnosed, then direct admission to a hospital coronary care unit is likely.

THE RAPID ACCESS CHEST PAIN CLINIC (RACPC)

These clinics (within hospitals) are designed to see patients for whom a diagnosis has not been established for their chest pain. A referral is made after basic testing has been done by the GP, including blood tests for full blood count (or 'FBC', the standard blood test showing haemoglobin levels and numbers of red blood cells, white blood cells and platelets), cholesterol levels and blood-glucose levels, a resting ECG, and possibly a chest X-ray if there was the possibility of heart failure.

A specialist will see the patient and a further examination and 'history taking' will be carried out. It is likely that an exercise ECG will be arranged.

The exercise ECG

This is also known as a treadmill ECG or a stress test. It is essentially an ECG performed on a patient while they walk on a treadmill or ride a bicycle. The treadmill is gradually increased in speed every two or three minutes and the gradient is increased. This simulates walking faster and faster uphill.

If stable angina is present then chest pain will occur and the test is stopped. It is also stopped if breathlessness occurs or if the person feels unwell or tired. Signs of ischaemia (as in Figure 17) will develop on the ECG in 85 per cent of cases with stable angina. If it takes a long time for the pain to develop (the test normally takes about 40 minutes), then doctors may diagnose mild stable angina and advise treatment.

If changes or pain occur rapidly, then further investigations are likely to be advised and arranged to determine the degree of myocardial ischaemia and to determine whether the patient is likely to need some form of revascularisation, whether that is by angioplasty (see Chapter 12), the insertion of a stent or even cardiac surgery to replace the diseased and narrowed coronary arteries.

It isn't necessarily angina – the differential diagnosis of chest pain

Common conditions that cause chest pain, and which may have to be eliminated (or confirmed) as part of the testing for heart disease, include the following:

Indigestion or heartburn

This is caused by acid from the stomach being squirted back upwards into the oesophagus (gullet). This tube is not equipped to deal with acid and it becomes irritated. It characteristically comes on after eating and can produce a very severe chest pain. A differentiating factor from angina is that it does not come on after exertion, whereas angina does.

Musculoskeletal chest-wall pain

This is usually from the straining of a muscle in the chest and there may be an obvious history of it. It tends to be a more localised pain than angina. It tends to be worse on movement and it is likely to be identifiable from the tenderness experienced on pressure.

Anxiety and hyperventilation

If you suffer an acute anxiety attack and start 'overbreathing', you may invoke chest pains and palpitations and simulate angina. The pains arise because overbreathing causes you to forcefully expel your carbon dioxide. This then causes a state of alkalosis, a shift in the normal pH (acidity measurement) of the blood. As a result of this there will be an alteration in calcium ionisation within the blood, which produces change in the sensations in the muscles and chest pain can occur. Once the overbreathing has stopped, the carbon dioxide level is restored and the alkalosis will go, as will the chest pain.

Pneumonia and pleurisy

Pneumonia is a severe chest infection. It does not usually cause any chest pain unless the covering of the lung (the pleura) is affected.

When the pleura is inflamed it will produce pain whenever it is stretched; this is pleurisy. Breathing in causes such stretching and the pain in pleurisy is typically whenever you take a deep breath. It also tends to be quite localised to one side of the chest. It does not produce tenderness when pressed from outside.

Pleurisy can also occur without an obvious underlying pneumonia, as a complication of various types of viral infections.

Pulmonary embolism

This is a potentially life-threatening condition. A pulmonary embolism (PE) is the name for a loose clot (embolus) from a deep-vein thrombosis (DVT) that lodges in a lung vessel. Thromboembolism is the name given to the pathological process that causes a blood clot to form in a vein in the first place. If the clot fragments, then the circulation will carry it round the body to lodge in a blood vessel in the lungs.

It typically produces a chest pain, rather like pleurisy, and the person may cough up blood. It is liable to occur in any state in which the blood is prone to clot. The oral contraceptive pill is an important example of how a drug may make the blood more likely to clot or produce a deep-vein thrombosis.

The combination of calf pain and chest pain are highly suggestive of a DVT with a pulmonary embolism and they require emergency treatment.

Gallstones and pancreatitis

Both of these conditions affect organs of the upper abdomen, but can produce pain radiating up into the chest.

Aortic disease

It is possible for the lining of the aorta to split. It causes excruciating pain and must be dealt with as an emergency, since emergency surgery may be needed.

The dissection of the lining causes two channels to exist in the aorta. One channel allows blood to flow through the vessel and the other causes blood to flow into the vessel wall. It occurs in two out of every 100,000 people, mainly in men between the ages of 40 and 70, but more commonly at the upper end of that age scale.

Pericarditis

As we have seen in Chapter 9, this is an inflammation of the sac that envelops the heart. The main symptoms are fever and chest pain, which can be sharp and incapacitating. The pain may be worse on deep inspiration or on swallowing or coughing, and should be dealt with as an emergency to exclude other conditions such as myocardial infarction.

Crush fracture

This is a painful condition caused by collapse of an osteoporotic vertebra in the spine. This is most common in elderly females and can produce severe back and chest pain.

Shingles

This is a condition caused by the varicella-zoster virus, the virus that causes chickenpox. After you have chickenpox, the virus stays in your body in a skin nerve. It may not cause problems for many years, but at a time when the body is perhaps a little below par, it flares up, causing pain along the course of that nerve. It also produces a rash like chickenpox in that area. It is commonest in people over the age of 50, although anyone who has had chickenpox is at risk. Unlike chickenpox, you can't catch shingles from someone who has it.

It is treatable and it is important to examine the skin if chest pain is experienced to exclude or confirm this condition.

Further investigations to be carried out

In the investigation of chest pain, in addition to resting and exercise ECGs, the following further investigations may need to be carried out to determine whether there is myocardial ischaemia resulting from coronary artery disease. These may be done in an outpatient clinic at an appointed time, but not on the same day as the rapid access chest pain clinic appointment.

Nuclear imaging

This is a very sophisticated test using certain radioactive nuclear isotopes that will accumulate in the heart tissue before quickly clearing from the body. There is no danger whatsoever from the radioactivity, which is minute and does not last long. Any traces are cleared in the urine. The isotopes will determine precisely any area of heart damage.

The isotopes used are usually thallium or technetium. They are given by injection into a vein. The different body tissues take them up at different amounts. The heart muscle will take them up if it has a good enough blood supply, but if it doesn't then they will not be taken up and they will not show when a scan is taken.

As with other tests to see if there is ischaemia on exertion, which is the feature of angina, the scan can be taken at rest and then again after exercise on a treadmill. The two scans are then compared.

Echocardiography

As mentioned in Chapter 8, an echocardiogram is a test using sound waves to build up a picture of the heart as it beats. It is done rather like a resting ECG, with the patient lying down whilst a transducer, which emits sound waves, is held against the chest. The echo from it produces a picture on a monitor, which shows the heart pumping and also shows the functioning of the valves. It will also show the way that the heart muscle is contracting. If it is ischaemic, then it will show up as poor contraction in that part of the heart.

A stress echocardiogram may also be done after the heart has been stimulated, as this may reveal changes in the way that the heart is pumping that are not apparent with an ordinary echocardiogram. The stress echocardiogram can be done with drugs or after a session on the treadmill.

Coronary angiogram

This is the most precise test, but it is an invasive technique that is not entirely without risk. It involves injecting a dye into the arterial system, which will outline the coronary arteries on a special X-ray. The possible risks are realised in one in a thousand cases and include:

- Irregular heart rhythm being provoked
- The coronary artery being damaged by the catheter
- The blood pressure dropping suddenly

- An allergic reaction to the dye
- A stroke being provoked
- The onset of myocardial infarction.

> **INDICATIONS OF THE NEED FOR CORONARY ANGIOGRAPHY**
>
> Not everyone with angina will need to have this test. It is mainly indicated if there is doubt about the diagnosis or if it is suspected that the person would benefit from angioplasty (see next chapter) or heart surgery. The following are the main indications for having one:
>
> - Angina experienced for the first time
> - Unstable angina
> - Aortic stenosis
> - Atypical chest pain, when other tests are normal
> - After an abnormal heart-stress test
> - You are to have surgery on your heart and you are at high risk of coronary artery disease
> - There is heart failure
> - There has been a recent heart attack.

The coronary angiography procedure has to be done in a special X-ray catheter laboratory. It involves inserting a catheter into an artery in the groin (or sometimes in the wrist) and passing it up into the heart and into the blocked area of the coronary arteries. This is done under X-ray control so that the catheter can be positioned exactly. Once it is in position, dye is injected which will show any blockages under X-ray. The whole process takes about 30–60 minutes. It is important to lie down for three hours afterwards, in order to prevent extensive bruising over the groin. A nurse or attendant will exert pressure over the area, since the catheter was inserted into an artery (arterial sites bleed more than venous ones).

If the coronary arteries are open and have good flow through them, as shown by the dye, then no further intervention is needed. If a blockage is found, then it can be dealt with by coronary angioplasty and stent insertion. This is called 'percutaneous coronary intervention' (PCI), which we shall deal with in the next chapter.

Treatment of angina

The whole aim of treatment is to prevent further episodes of pain, or to offer the means to control them. In addition, the aim is to do all that is possible to reduce the risk of having a heart attack. The following treatments are relevant:

Lifestyle change

This is essential if there are risk factors that can be modified. Smoking should be stopped. If the individual is overweight then dietary advice should be given and a concerted effort made to reduce the weight to a safe limit. And daily exercise should be taken, since there is good evidence that this reduces the risk of having a myocardial infarction.

Drug treatment

We have an array of invaluable drugs that can make life bearable and render the condition manageable.

> **KEY POINTS**
>
> Three types of drug may be prescribed in the treatment of angina:
>
> - Antiplatelet drugs, including aspirin, to stop blood clots forming
> - Antianginals – to reduce the pain of angina
> - Statins – to reduce cholesterol.

Antiplatelet drugs

There are two main ones, aspirin and clopidogrel:

Aspirin

Over the years this drug has proven to be of inestimable value in reducing the risk of strokes, heart attacks and various types of cancer.[15] It is an antiplatelet drug, which means that it stops platelets, the very smallest blood cells, from sticking together to produce a blood clot. It is usually prescribed in a daily dose of 75 mg, indefinitely, and it can save lives.

Unfortunately, not everyone can take aspirin, including, of course, anyone who is allergic to it. It cannot be used by those with a gastric ulcer or with a tendency to a bleeding disorder. In some cases of dyspepsia, however, another drug that protects the stomach may be given at the same time.

> ### THE LIFE OF A PLATELET
>
> A platelet lives for only about ten days, and aspirin will cause it to lose its ability to clot for the duration of its life. This means that after you take an aspirin tablet, your platelets will be less sticky than they were before you took the aspirin, and the effect will persist for a week.

Clopidogrel

This is an alternative to aspirin for those patients who cannot tolerate it, or who are allergic to it. It is not so likely to upset the stomach.

Antianginals

There are several types that may be used, including beta blockers, calcium channel blockers and nitrates:

Beta blockers

These are the first line and are generally prescribed as soon as coronary heart disease is suspected. They are called this because they block special receptors found in heart muscles, lungs, arteries and smooth muscle (which are all part of the sympathetic nervous system that we looked at in Chapter 4). By blocking these receptors they slow down the heart and they reduce the blood pressure, which together allow the heart to tolerate more exertion without invoking angina.

Some beta blockers are more selective than others, in that they target predominantly the cardiovascular beta receptors, rather than the respiratory ones. Some people cannot take the ones that target respiratory receptors, e.g. if they suffer from asthma, since the beta blocker could provoke an asthma attack.

Other side effects include vivid dreams, cold extremities, pins and needles in the hands and feet, muscle heaviness in the legs and sexual difficulties including loss of libido and erectile dysfunction.

Common beta blockers are propranolol, acebutolol, bisoprolol, atenolol, metoprolol and oxprenolol.

Calcium channel blockers

These block the flow of calcium into muscle cells in the blood vessel walls, as we saw in Chapter 4. This has the effect of dilating the coronary arteries, but they do not slow the heart as beta blockers do. They can be used in combination with beta blockers or with the third group of drugs, the nitrates.

The most commonly prescribed channel blockers are amlodipine in a daily dose or diltiazem in a dose twice a day. Other ones are felodipine, nifedipine, nicardipine and isradipine. Their potential side effects are headaches, dizziness, ankle swelling and constipation.

Nitrates

These are the oldest effective treatment for angina. They cause dilatation of arteries and veins throughout the whole body. This is obviously of benefit to the heart during an anginal attack, but it can produce side effects elsewhere. The commonest side effect complained of is headache, since the blood vessels in the scalp and brain can dilate, stretching the vessel walls and stimulating pain sensors in them.

Nitrates work remarkably quickly, literally within seconds, and most anginal attacks can be aborted within five minutes of sucking a small glyceryl trinitrate (GTN) tablet, or after applying a nitrolingual spray under the tongue.

In addition to these two methods, there are other longer-lasting nitrates that may be given in order to prevent angina. Some work by slow absorption when left under the inner lip, and others can be given as patches. Isosorbide dinitrate and isosorbide mononitrate are longer-lasting nitrates that can be taken as tablets or capsules.

> **KEY POINT**
>
> During an angina attack you can take a second dose of GTN or nitrolingual spray, but if there is no relief after ten minutes then help should be sought urgently.

Statins

These are drugs that may be given to reduce lipids (which we covered in Chapter 10) in the blood. Statins reduce mortality rates by about one-third so they are invaluable as drugs. They are the drugs of first choice in reducing cholesterol levels and can in fact reduce the level by up to 40 per cent. They do this by reducing the production of cholesterol in the liver.

Statins (or HMG-CoA reductase inhibitors, to give them their full name) have been used for several years to reduce cholesterol levels. They work by inhibiting the enzyme HMG-CoA reductase, which is involved in cholesterol synthesis. The statins work to reduce the level of the enzyme in the liver, which will in turn result in a decrease in the level of cholesterol. They also increase the synthesis of LDL receptors, which helps them to clear low-density lipoproteins from the blood.

Some people react to statins and may develop muscle cramps or an inflammatory condition of the muscles called a myopathy, which at its extreme form can cause a breakdown in muscle tissue, called rhabdomyolysis. Nerve damage is also a rare possibility. Having said that, most people tolerate statins and if one statin produces side effects then another in the group may be tolerated well.

Commonly used statins are atorvastatin, fluvastatin, pravastatin, simvastatin and rosuvastatin.

Fibrates

These are another group of drugs that are often used in combination with statins if there is difficulty in reducing both cholesterol and triglyceride levels (triglycerides are the other blood lipids we looked at in Chapter 10). Commonly used fibrates are bezafibrate, ciprofibrate and fenofibrate.

The side effects of fibrates, particularly when used in conjunction with statins, include hair loss and muscular problems, including a condition called myositis, when the muscles become inflamed. They can also cause gastro-intestinal problems, and (rarely) pancreatitis and alteration of liver function.

Newer drugs

- *Ivabradine*: effective at slowing the heart, like beta blockers, but less likely to produce side effects.

- *Ranolazine*: often used if other antianginals have not worked adequately. Helps to reduce the effect of ischaemia in the heart muscle.

Other treatments

Angioplasty, stent insertion and cardiac surgery will be considered in the next chapter.

Chapter 12

Heart attacks – what happens

> **KEY POINTS**
>
> - About 240,000 people have a heart attack in England and Wales every year.
> - 50 per cent of those who die from a heart attack do so within the first hour.
> - Death is commonly due to an abnormal rhythm being provoked.
> - The risk of death declines hour by hour.
> - Emergency treatment is essential, including the immediate use of aspirin and access to a defibrillator if necessary.
> - If a coronary artery is blocked for longer than 5–10 minutes, the area of myocardium (heart muscle) supplied by it will die. This is a myocardial infarction.
> - Most complications occur within the first 48 hours post infarction.

If you develop sudden severe chest pain that makes you feel clammy and nauseated, you may be having a heart attack. If you have a history of angina and have a supply of GTN tablets or a nitrolingual spray, then try one, then repeat after five minutes. If there is no improvement then, call for medical aid. If you have never had angina and experience such a pain, call for medical aid immediately.

Emergency care

This may be in the form of a GP rushing to see you, or more probably an ambulance team of paramedics being dispatched to see you. They will assess you as quickly as possible, by asking some questions and performing an examination and doing an ECG, using chest leads.

The whole aim is to make an initial assessment and stabilise your medical condition at that moment, probably inside the ambulance, before taking you to hospital.

Oxygen

This will be given by face mask.

Intravenous canula

This is a small tube (with a tap), which will be inserted into a vein in the arm or the back of the wrist. This will permit drugs to be delivered direct into the bloodstream.

Pain relief

A strong drug such as morphine may be given to alleviate pain. It may be combined with another drug to reduce nausea.

Aspirin

It is usual to give 300 mg of aspirin in a single tablet to start treating any clot that may at that very moment be blocking a coronary artery. The aspirin starts to work instantly and blocks the stickiness of platelets that may otherwise aggregate on an already developed small clot.

Irregular heart rhythms

These are called arrhythmias. If there are any which are life threatening, they will be treated immediately with drugs.

Cardiac arrest

If the heart has stopped, a defibrillator may be used to restart it.

In hospital

Once in hospital you are assessed again. It is likely that you will be diagnosed as having acute coronary syndrome (ACS). This is the working diagnosis, which will be modified and refined as tests are performed.

Acute coronary syndrome

This means that myocardial ischaemia is causing symptoms of chest pain and other symptoms and signs, including possibly heart rhythm abnormalities, alterations in blood pressure and heart failure. There are three main possibilities:

- *Unstable angina* – this is severe chest pain associated with either no alteration in the ECG or only temporary ST elevation. No rise in enzyme levels are found, so no damage to the heart muscle is assumed.

- *NSTEMI* – this means non-ST elevation myocardial infarction. With this condition the arterial supply is only partially blocked off, so only part of the heart muscle is damaged. The ECG will, as with unstable angina, only show temporary changes. There will be enzyme changes, indicating some damage to heart tissue.

- *STEMI* – this means ST elevation myocardial infarction, which means the arterial supply to the whole thickness of part of the heart muscle is completely blocked off. There will be enzyme changes indicating heart muscle damage.

The importance of differentiating them is because they require different treatments. STEMI requires clot-busting treatment, and NSTEMI and unstable angina do not.

Initial management

The patient will be monitored with a continuous ECG monitor, so that changes in the clinical picture can be picked up immediately. If dangerous heart rhythms show up, they can be treated, with a defibrillator if necessary. Treatment may also include oxygen delivery, pain relief with diamophine (heroin), anti-nausea drugs and aspirin.

Further investigation to determine exactly what has happened to the heart will include:

- Physical examination to elicit any murmurs, determine the state of the blood pressure, and find any evidence of heart failure.

- ECG (see box below).
- Chest X-ray – to assess the size of the heart and detect any heart failure.
- Blood tests – to measure blood sugar levels, biochemical markers (enzymes) of heart damage and lipid levels.

> **ECG CHANGES IN ACUTE CORONARY SYNDROME**
>
> There are a number of tests that can tell if the heart muscle is damaged. The ECG is the main test to differentiate the types of myocardial infarction, and it is combined with blood tests to measure cardiac troponin levels over several days.
>
> If the heart muscle is damaged, it may not conduct sufficient electricity, so this will produce changes on the ECG, which measures the electrical activity of the heart muscle. If the whole thickness of the heart muscle is infarcted, then that part will not conduct electricity at all. So, the ECG being recorded at the lead that is 'looking at' that part of the heart will not see any activity from that part of the muscle. Effectively, it is like looking through a hole and it will register or 'see' the activity in the muscle of the heart directly opposite it. That is how changes are produced on the ECG.
>
> The most significant change is the ST change. It may be elevated from the neutral line, because instead of seeing normal activity, you see the electrical impulse moving away from the part of the heart opposite the damaged area. Thus it seems to be elevated upwards on the ECG tracing.

The leads that show the change can thus pinpoint where the myocardial infarction takes place. For example:

- Anterior infarction shows as ST elevation and Q waves in chest leads V1–V5.
- Inferior infarction shows in leads II, III and aVF.

After a myocardial infarction there may be other permanent signs of damage on the ECG. A Q wave indicates past myocardial infarction. The majority of STEMI patients will go on to develop Q waves.

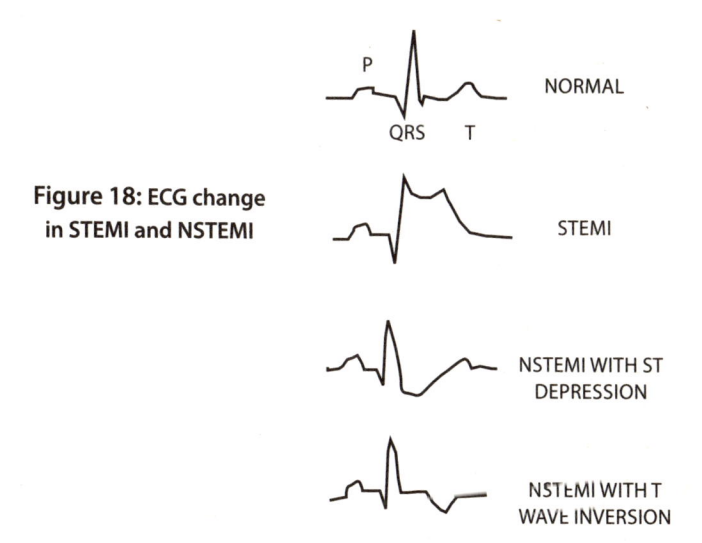

Figure 18: ECG change in STEMI and NSTEMI

Biochemical markers of myocardial damage

Essentially, these are enzymes that leach out of damaged heart muscle and which can be found in elevated levels in the blood. Creatine kinase (CK) levels rise four to eight hours after STEMI and fall to normal in three to four days. Troponin T (TnT) and troponin

I (TnI) are very sensitive markers – they rise after three hours and stay elevated for up to 14 days. These markers can therefore be very useful if investigations are being done days after an event, as is the case with a silent myocardial infarction, when the patient felt unwell, but without the severe chest pain normally associated with a myocardial infarction.

> **KEY POINTS**
>
> - The annual incidence of NSTEMI hospital admissions is about three per thousand members of the population.[16]
> - It is harder to diagnose NSTEMI than STEMI.

The diagnostic process

We can summarise the process in Figure 19, which shows how the three conditions (unstable angina, NSTEMI or STEMI) are diagnosed:

Reperfusion

This is the name given to the process of opening up blocked arteries to restore blood flow. The earlier this is done the better, in order to limit damage to the heart muscle and to preserve the function of the heart as a pump.

There are two ways that this can be done:

- *Clot-busting* – with drugs called thrombolytics.
- *Percutaneous coronary intervention (PCI)* – which involves reopening an artery with a balloon and inserting a stent to keep that artery open.

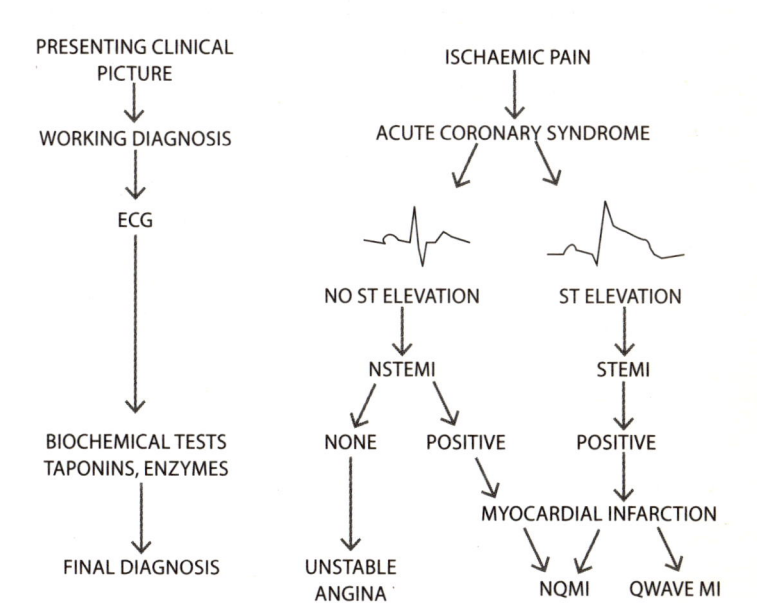

Figure 19: The diagnostic process in acute coronary syndrome

Clot-busting

This is the use of a thrombolytic (also known as fibrinoltytic) drug to break up a blood clot. It is only given if there is evidence of STEMI myocardial infarction – that is, if the full thickness of the heart muscle is damaged. There is a time limit, however, and that is 12 hours. Some studies suggest that if there is definite evidence at presentation, then a thrombolytic drug should be given straight away by the paramedics in the ambulance. The usual clot-buster is called streptokinase, and it is given by intravenous infusion through a drip. Others are alteplase, reteplase and tenecteplase. An anticoagulant called herapin is sometimes given for a couple of days in combination with the clot-buster.

Clot-busting is not without risk, so it should not be given to people who have had a stroke or a major bleed. Possible side effects include nausea and vomiting, increased risk of bleeding and, especially with streptokinase, an allergic reaction.

Percutaneous coronary intervention

This is the procedure known as a primary angioplasty, and it is the preferred method of treatment if it can be performed within 90 minutes of the time that the patient has received thombolysis. It can be carried out up to four hours after the myocardial infarction.

It is used to treat angina and also to clear a blockage after a myocardial infarction. With angina it can be a planned procedure, and with STEMI it can be carried out as an emergency treatment.

It usually takes between 30 minutes and two hours and is done with continuous X-ray monitoring in a special catheter lab. Because it is done with an angiogram, it is necessary to insert dye into the bloodstream so it involves numbing an area of skin over an artery, either at the wrist or the groin, and inserting a canula. Then a fine hollow catheter with a balloon on its tip (which in turn is surrounded by a stent) is inserted up the artery and through the heart to the opening that feeds into the coronary arteries. Dye is then injected into the coronary arteries to outline the blockage.

The patient may be aware of this and feel a flush as the dye goes through the system.

The catheter is then advanced up to the blockage and the balloon is inflated. This will compress the blockage caused by the fatty plaques of atheroma and will widen the artery as it is inflated.

The stent, basically a cylindrical tube of stainless steel mesh, is expanded with the balloon and will remain in place once the balloon is deflated and withdrawn. It stays in position and keeps the blood vessel open.

After the procedure the catheter is removed and pressure is maintained over the entrance to the artery to prevent bleeding. Sometimes a special plug called an angioseal will be used to stop further bleeding and bruising.

In the majority of cases there are no problems, but if chest pain occurs afterwards then the medical staff should be alerted.

Post procedure

If the angioplasty had been planned for angina control, then the patient may be able to go home the same day or the day after the procedure. If it was done after a myocardial infarction, then there is likely to be a need for more stabilisation with medication and the patient will remain in hospital.

For the next week there should be no lifting or exertion. If it was a planned procedure then light work may be possible after a few days. If it was after a myocardial infarction then several weeks, rest may be required and advised.

KEY POINTS

- The results from over ten randomised trials comparing PCI with thrombolysis suggest that PCI is the treatment of choice
- PCI patients are less likely to have a further myocardial infarction than thrombolytic patients.
- PCI is less likely to cause haemorrhage than thrombolysis.

COMPLICATIONS OF A MYOCARDIAL INFARCTION

There are several complications of such heart attacks, all of which need to be investigated and treated vigorously:

- Abnormal rhythms (arrhythmias).
- Cardiac arrest – the heart stops and must be restarted immediately.
- Cardiogenic shock – multiple organs can start to fail because the heart is not able to adequately supply them with blood.
- Cardiac rupture – after the previous two complications, both of which can lead to death, this is the commonest cause of fatality. It occurs in 10 per cent of cases, usually between days five to ten as the damaged heart muscle is healing and rupture can take place through the weakened muscle.
- Heart failure – the heart attack may have weakened the heart and compromised its ability to function properly as a pump. This may need ongoing medication.
- Rupture of papillary muscles – these are muscles inside the heart which operate the heart valves. This can lead to incompetence of the valve and rapid heart failure.
- Pericarditis – inflammation of the sac that contains the heart. This occurs in 20 per cent of patients within 24 to 72 hours after the event and causes further tight chest pain. It is usually self-limiting, meaning that it settles spontaneously.

> ### SUDDEN CARDIAC ARREST (SCA)
>
> - This is an abrupt loss of pulse and consciousness caused by an unexpected failure in the heart's ability to maintain a circulation of blood to the brain and body.
> - It is usually caused by life-threatening arrhythmias, in turn caused by a problem in the heart's electrical conducting system.
> - The arrhythmia causing this is usually ventricular fibrillation.
> - The sudden cardiac arrest victim first loses his or her pulse, then consciousness, then stops breathing. All of this happens within seconds.
> - About 100,000 people die from sudden cardiac arrest every year in the UK.
> - Without immediate treatment, 90–95 per cent of SCA victims will die.
> - Until a defibrillator is available, life can be maintained by effective cardiopulmonary resuscitation, known as CPR.
> - The definitive treatment is defibrillation – this involves using a machine called a defibrillator to deliver an electric current to the chest, which 'shocks' the heart into resuming a normal rhythm. This 'shock' must be delivered within minutes of the arrest to successfully prevent death.

Irregular hearts

After a myocardial infarction some patients may develop arrhythmias (irregularities of the heart). Stabilising them is one of the mainstays of ongoing treatment.

Beta blockers are used by many cardiologists to slow the heart and reduce the risk of irregularities, since very often the heart rate is inclined to increase following an infarction. Not everyone can take beta blockers, however, and if there is any evidence of heart block (which we shall look at in Chapter 14) then it is absolutely contraindicated, because it could slow the heart too much and make the condition worse.

ACE inhibitors

Every patient, after having received aspirin, beta blockers and reperfusion, should receive an ACE inhibitor (normally used to treat high blood pressure) within 24 hours of the myocardial infarction. This is of immense benefit in preventing reinfarction and heart failure.

The uncomplicated myocardial infarction

Although we have talked about the complications that can occur after a myocardial infarction, a great many people have an uncomplicated recovery. Most problems tend to occur in the first 48 hours, but thereafter recovery is generally smooth.

The area of heart muscle that is infarcted will be repaired with fibrous tissue to produce a scar. This will take six to eight weeks. If the area affected has been relatively small, there should be a complete return to normal life.

If the area affected has been larger, then the scar tissue in that area may be less functional than heart muscle, so it may impair the pump action of the heart. Some degree of heart failure may be the result, but various drugs may be used to help that, as we shall see in Chapter 13.

Drugs on discharge from hospital

A lot of people are surprised at the number of drugs that they are discharged from hospital with. They may have gone from taking nothing at all to taking three or four different types of drugs. They are important, however, and will all be given to maintain health and to reduce the risk of having another heart attack. The drugs given will likely be among the following types:

Antiplatelet drugs

As we have seen, these are usually aspirin or clopidogrel, both of which work to stop platelets sticking together to form a clot in the blood.

Beta blockers

Used to block adrenaline and noradrenaline receptors in the heart and in blood vessels, which in turn slows the heart and reduces the risk of another heart attack. They have been shown to reduce the death rate after heart attacks.

ACE inhibitors or angiotensin receptor blockers (ARBs)

Amazingly successful drugs used to treat or prevent heart failure and reduce the risk of having a further heart attack.

Diuretics

These may be given to make the person pass more urine if there has been some heart failure, because they remove fluid from areas where it has accumulated during the failure, such as the lungs and the lower limbs. The most commonly prescribed of these is furosemide.

Statins

As we have seen, these are drugs used to reduce bad cholesterol.

Chapter 13

Managing heart failure

As we discussed in Chapter 6, heart failure is a complex problem that occurs when the heart fails to meet the demands of the body. It is not always easy to diagnose the exact type of heart failure on simple clinical grounds and special tests are therefore often needed.

The range of symptoms

The following are the main symptoms of heart failure:

Breathlessness

You tend to feel breathless in situations that you would not expect to. There may be a gradually increasing tendency to be breathless on slight exertion, such as going up stairs. It can then become more severe and occur even at rest. If this is the case, then it needs to be differentiated from other conditions, such as asthma or emphysema.

Breathlessness lying flat

This is significant and it may be that you have to use four or more pillows at night to prevent the breathlessness. If such severe breathlessness occurs it is important to tell your doctor.

Oedema (ankle swelling)

There are lots of conditions that may cause swelling of the ankles. Air travel or long train journeys can produce it, as can standing for long periods. Women may retain fluid before periods. All of these conditions are quite normal. In heart failure, however, the swelling is likely to be very marked, getting worse as the day goes by, but tending to go down while at rest overnight. A characteristic sign is 'pitting oedema', which means that if the swelling is pressed with a finger and thumb, then a pit is left in the skin after it has been released.

Nocturia

This is the passage of urine at night, more than you are typically used to. Here again, there are several other conditions that may be stimulating the bladder. Men in particular may suffer from prostate problems. If in doubt, have it checked.

Fatigue

This is almost always the case. The fact is that the heart is not managing to maintain an adequate circulation, so when it is asked to do any extra work, even in normal tasks, then it will struggle to do so. The effect is that the body is not supplied with enough oxygen for its needs and fatigue will result.

Chest pain

This can occur if there is underlying myocardial ischaemia from coronary artery disease. It can be a vicious circle, because the weakened heart muscle may be more susceptible to ischaemia and therefore heart failure may further deprive it of oxygen, and chest pain may be the result.

Palpitations

The heart may be deprived of oxygen through heart failure and may speed up to try to push more blood round the circulation. The sensation of palpitations or speeding up of the heart may be apparent.

Other symptoms

These might be constipation, anorexia, bloating of the stomach, confusion, insomnia or poor sleep.

Physical signs the doctor will look for

The doctor will look for the following:

Oedema

This may be limited to pitting oedema in the ankles, but the more severe the failure the greater the degree of oedema, so the swelling may extend up past the knees to the thighs. In very severe failure it can even spread up to the abdominal wall. Impressions of clothing may be apparent, such as the tops of socks or the belt line.

Hepatomegaly

This means enlargement of the liver. If the right side of the heart is struggling, there will be a back-pressure effect on the circulation taking blood back to the heart. The liver, being the major organ that blood flows through on its way back to the heart, may then swell. The doctor will assess this by examining the abdomen to feel for a liver edge, and by percussion, which involves tapping the back of one finger of the flat hand on the abdomen, with a finger of the other hand.

Pulmonary oedema

This is accumulation of fluid within the lungs. The doctor will listen to the chest for sounds of fluid in the small airways. It is a sign of left-sided heart failure.

Raised JVP

This stands for jugular venous pressure, which is a rise in pressure in the jugular vein, one of the main neck veins. In right-sided heart failure the neck veins may appear congested and the doctor may see a small pulsation in the jugular vein. This indicates back pressure from the right side of the heart.

Pinpointing the problem

The following investigations may be needed to get a more accurate picture of the condition:

Blood tests

The main test is called BNP, which stands for brain natriuretic peptide, a protein that is released by the ventricles of the heart into the blood when they are overstretched.

It is therefore a highly sensitive blood test for a protein level that is raised in heart failure. A normal result usually indicates that the person has another reason for their symptoms. Generally speaking, the higher the level, the more severe the heart failure.

Other standard biochemical blood tests measuring kidney function, blood sugar levels, full blood counts, thyroid function and lipids may also be asked for.

ECG

A full 12-lead ECG will be carried out to look for irregularity of the heart rhythm or evidence of myocardial ischaemia, or other changes that may be significant.

CXR

A chest X-ray may indicate enlargement of the heart or evidence of pulmonary oedema.

Echocardiogram

This is a good test, since sound waves bouncing off the heart and its ventricles and valves will give a visual image of how the heart is functioning. One of the most important pieces of information that can be obtained from this investigation is the function of the left ventricle.

A specific measurement called the left ventricular ejection fraction (LVEF) is often given. This is an estimate of how much of the blood that enters the left ventricle is pumped out when the heart muscle contracts. It is expressed as a percentage.

In a healthy heart, about 60 per cent of the blood entering the left ventricle is pumped out when the heart muscle contracts. A value of less than 40 per cent indicates that your heart is not pumping normally, that there is heart failure.

If the diagnosis is still in doubt after the tests above have been carried out, or if there is a suggestion of further intensive treatment, possibly including surgery, then more specialised investigations such as the following may be helpful:

Exercise test

This is the stress test that we considered earlier in the book. It can be done on a treadmill or a bicycle, and may be combined with an oxygen consumption test to determine how much oxygen you are using.

Nuclear imaging

Using a radioactive tracer injected into the bloodstream (as we already saw in Chapter 11), the uptake of the tracer by the heart muscle will give an image of the heart and the way that it functions with each beat.

Angiography

As indicated in the last chapter, this specialised X-ray technique may be applied in order to assess the coronary arteries, especially if surgery is a possibility.

MRI

MRI stands for magnetic resonance imaging. It is an investigation that uses magnetism, ultrasound and computerised technology to build up multiple images of the inside of the body. This may show the tissues and any derangement of them in surprising detail.

It can be an alarming investigation for people who are prone to claustrophobia, since with some scanners it necessitates being advanced through a large tunnel-like apparatus.

> ### THE SEVERITY OF HEART FAILURE
>
> There are various classifications for the severity of heart failure. One such is the New York Heart Association (NYHA) Classification.
>
> - Class I – no limitation of activity.
> - Class II – slight limitation, producing symptoms on ordinary activity, e.g. climbing stairs.
> - Class III – marked limitation, producing symptoms on minimal levels of exertion, e.g. dressing.
> - Class IV – symptoms present at rest.

Treatment of heart failure

The whole aim of treatment is to improve the health of the individual with heart failure, to reduce symptoms and to reduce deterioration of the condition. An appropriate combination of the following treatments will be offered:

Lifestyle change

This may sound simplistic, but it is often crucial and immensely beneficial. If you smoke, then stopping smoking can reduce symptoms, as can stopping drinking excess alcohol. Increasing exercise and reducing weight may also have a huge impact.

Your hospital department may include you in a rehabilitation programme of diet, exercise and support.

Medical treatment

There are a large number of drugs that may be beneficial. If the cause of the heart failure is another condition, such as thyroid disease, then treating the thyroid (for example) may solve or go a long way to improving the heart failure.

Most patients with left ventricular systolic dysfunction (LVSD), a weak heart, or with diastolic heart failure, a stiff heart, will benefit from a combination of the following drugs (you can look back at Chapter 4 if you want a reminder about how these various drugs are employed to good effect on the sympathetic nervous system and the renin-angiotensin-aldosterone system):

Diuretics

These are water pills that make you pass more urine, which can help with breathlessness, high blood pressure and swelling of the ankles and lower extremities. There are several that may be used, but bendroflumethiazide (in mild cases), furosemide and bumetanide are the most common.

The thiazide diuretics, of which bendroflumethiazide is one, tend to cause you to lose potassium, so this needs to be monitored by the doctor, because potassium is an important element in the body. It is involved in the electrical conduction system of the heart and either high levels, known as hyperkalaemia, or low levels, known as hypokalaemia, can result in serious irregularities of the heart.

ACE inhibitors

These are angiotensin-converting-enzyme inhibitors. As we saw in Chapter 4, they work by dilating the blood vessels to reduce blood pressure and enhance blood flow. They are regarded as the most important drugs in heart failure and they make a dramatic difference on quality of life and reduce the risk of hospitalisation. They do undoubtedly improve life expectancy for people with heart failure. The most commonly used ones are lisinopril, perindopril, captopril, ramipril and enalapril.

ACE inhibitors do have some side effects, the most troublesome one being a dry irritant cough. They can also cause:

- Dizziness
- Low blood pressure
- Disordered kidney function
- Altered potassium levels
- Increased ankle swelling.

The dizziness may be the result of the ACE inhibitors lowering blood pressure too much, so the use of a diuretic at the same time as the ACE inhibitor can make any resultant swelling less problematic.

Because of the potential for ACE inhibitors to alter kidney function and potassium or sodium levels, it is important to have regular blood tests of those. Both sodium and potassium are important 'electrolytes' in the body, which means that they are substances that 'ionise' in the body fluids. Sodium is the main electrolyte in the blood and in the extracellular fluids, and is involved in fluid balance and blood pressure control.

Beta blockers

These are also generally indicated for most patients with LVSD heart failure. They are called beta blockers because they block certain hormone receptors found in heart muscles, lungs, arteries and smooth muscle, which are all part of the sympathetic nervous system we looked at in Chapter 4. By blocking these receptors they slow down the heart and reduce the blood pressure. This in turn allows the heart to tolerate more exertion without invoking angina. Not everyone, however, can take all types of beta blockers (for a reminder about their possible side effects, turn back to Chapter 11).

ARBs

Angiotensin receptor blockers (ARBs) work in a similar way to ACE inhibitors by widening blood vessels and reducing blood pressure. They may be prescribed instead of ACE inhibitors because they do not usually cause a cough.

Commonly used ARBs include candesartan, losartan, telmisartan and valsartan. They do also have side effects, including low blood pressure, which may cause dizziness, and they may cause high levels of potassium in the blood. It is for this reason that your doctor will carry out regular blood tests to monitor potassium levels.

Although ARBs do not cause coughs, and may therefore be more acceptable to take for some people, they may not be quite as effective as ACE inhibitors in the control of heart failure.

For some patients with severe heart failure who are unable to take aldosterone antagonists (see below), then an ARB may be used in addition to an ACE inhibitor.

Ivabradine

This drug slows the heart down. It is useful if the heart is beating too fast, but it should only be given if the rhythm is normal. It can be used as an alternative to beta blockers if the latter cannot be tolerated.

Aldosterone antagonists

These diuretics may be added in if the heart failure is not being adequately controlled by an appropriate combination of the above drugs. They work in a similar way to other diuretics, in that they increase urine production. They can dramatically improve heart failure by reducing scarring of the heart muscle but they can also cause potassium levels to rise, so once again your doctor will monitor this.

Nitrates

You may recall from Chapter 11 that these are the oldest treatment we have for angina, and that they have had a long-standing place in the treatment of heart failure. Although many of the newer drugs are replacing them, they still have a place in heart failure treatment if people are unable to take ACE inhibitors or ARBs for whatever reason.

The drug hydralazine may be prescribed in combination with the nitrates, as this combination causes the blood vessels to dilate, which in turn improves blood flow.

Digoxin

This is another one of our oldest effective drugs in cardiology. It is a type of drug called a cardiac glycoside, a purified drug that was first extracted from the foxglove plant *Digitalis lanata*. It was discovered in 1785 by William Withering (1741–1799), a Shropshire physician, after he had noted that an old woman who practised herbal medicine used a concoction for treating dropsy, which was the then name for heart failure. She achieved dramatic results and he analysed her concoction of 20 ingredients to work out that digitalis was the active beneficial agent.

Digoxin increases the strength of heart contractions and slows the heart down.

Anticoagulants

These drugs thin the blood to prevent it from coagulating. They may be prescribed for patients at risk of atrial fibrillation, i.e. of developing a blood clot that could break off and cause a stroke.

Warfarin has been the main oral anticoagulant until recently. Taking it necessitates having a regular blood test called an INR (international normalised ratio) to monitor the level of anticoagulation that has been achieved. The daily dosage can then be adjusted according to the findings of the local anticoagulant clinic (which could be the local hospital, GP surgery or even a pharmacy) doing the monitoring.

More recently, the National Institute for Health and Care Excellence (NICE) have approved two other oral anticoagulants, dabigatran and rivaroxaban, for use in the treatment of patients with atrial fibrillation, in order to reduce their risk of stroke. They both work in similar ways to warfarin, but they have the advantage of not having to have regular monitoring and dosage adjustment.

Antiplatelet agents

As we have seen, aspirin or clopidogrel may be prescribed to reduce the risk of having a stroke, or they may be given to patients with known coronary artery disease.

Calcium channel blockers

Again, as we have already seen, these can help in the treatment of heart failure as they cause dilation of blood vessels by blocking the flow of calcium into muscle cells.

Devices

There are various devices that may be helpful to support the heart in patients with heart failure, either to control the heart rate or the heart rhythm. We shall consider these and other treatments for irregular hearts in the next chapter.

Surgical treatment

As we shall see in the next chapter, if a device is to be used then a cardiac surgeon may have to be involved in the implantation of a pacemaker box. Other surgical treatments for heart failure include the following:

Valve surgery

If the cause of the heart failure is a faulty heart valve, then it may be possible to operate to improve your condition. There are two types of valve surgery:

- Valve repair
- Valve replacement.

With open surgery, the surgeon opens up the chest by making a large incision through the breastbone to expose the heart and the aorta. A heart-lung machine or bypass pump will then do the job of the heart while it is stopped during the operation.

Minimally invasive surgery for less serious valve conditions may be carried out through a 'keyhole', via a catheter being inserted through the skin.

Valve repair

This is usually carried out on the mitral and tricuspid valves. There are two main techniques:

- Ring annuloplasty – in which the circle round the valve is repaired by inserting and sewing a ring of plastic or tissue around the valve.

- Valve repair in which one or more of the valve cusps is rebuilt.

Valve replacement

This is the total replacement of a valve that is too damaged to repair, and is mainly used to replace the aortic valve. There are three types of valve replacement:

- *Mechanical valve* – these are made of metal, usually steel or titanium, or a ceramic material. They last a long time, but there is a risk of clot formation, so either an anticoagulant or an antiplatelet agent like aspirin will have to be taken for the rest of the patient's life.

- *Tissue valve* – from human or animal tissue. Generally, these will last 10–15 years, but the necessity of having a blood-thinning drug is not so great.

- *Ross procedure* – this involves replacing the patient's aortic valve with their own pulmonary valve, then replacing the pulmonary with an artificial-tissue or human-donor valve. This procedure may be used in children, because the 'new' aortic valve (actually their own pulmonary valve) may then continue to grow as the heart grows. Again, blood-thinning agents may not be required.

Surgery for coronary artery disease

We already covered the used of angioplasty and stent insertion in the last chapter.

Coronary artery bypass graft surgery

This is sometimes referred to as CABG. If the patient's coronary arteries are significantly narrowed or blocked, then they can be replaced with veins removed from the legs. This does no harm to the legs since they are superficial veins (veins close to the surface of the body used for cooling rather than primary blood circulation) that are used and the legs have sufficient deep veins that will continue to do the work needed to circulate blood around the legs.

Since the veins have one-way valves, they have to be reversed, so that the valves cease to function. One, two, three or four coronary arteries can be replaced, hence one can have a double, triple or quadruple CABG.

This is a major surgical procedure, yet it is so commonly carried out that surgeons are highly proficient in it and most patients suffer no problems. It usually dramatically improves angina and may help a patient with heart failure, since the myocardium starts to get an adequate supply of oxygen.

Aneurysmectomy

A ventricular aneurysm, a ballooning out of the ventricle wall after a myocardial infarction, is a potential cause of heart failure. It is possible that the aneurysm could be removed and the weakness improved, thereby alleviating heart failure in such patients.

Heart transplantation

The first successful heart transplantation was performed by Dr Christiaan Barnard in Cape Town in South Africa in 1967.

It is an operation that is performed for end-stage heart failure when other treatments have been unsuccessful, and it involves replacing the heart of the patient with that of a donor. The operation takes about 4–6 hours and hospital care is needed for about another 4–6 weeks.

It is important to appreciate that a heart transplant will not alter the recipient in any way, as the personality of the individual is not associated with the heart, as the ancients believed.

> **KEY POINT**
>
> In 2012 there were 145 heart transplants and 191 joint heart and lung transplants at seven hospitals in the UK.

Chapter 14

Irregular hearts

A normal heart beats in regular fashion, but a heart experiencing problems can be irregular in one of two ways:

- In rhythm
- In rate.

An irregular heartbeat is called an arrhythmia. This means that the heart is not beating with a regular rhythm, so there may be a number of fast beats followed by slow ones, or any number of other combinations.

An irregular heart rate means that the heart is beating an abnormal rate of beats per minute. The normal heart rate is 50–100 beats per minute. A slow heart rate is called a bradycardia. A fast heart rate is called a tachycardia.

Arrhythmias can occur at a slow heart rate, when they are called bradyarrhythmias, and they can occur at fast heart rates, when they are called tachyarrhythmias.

Symptoms of arrhythmias

When the heart is beating irregularly there are a number of symptoms that may be experienced:

Palpitations

This is the commonest symptom. It means having an awareness of the heart beating inside the chest. It may be a forceful, unpleasant hammering, or it may be a sensation of the heart beating very fast. There may even be the sensation of having missed a beat.

Shortness of breath

This is quite common if the heart is beating so fast and irregularly that it is not filling up adequately.

Dizziness or faintness

Again, if the heart is beating very fast and not filling up adequately, then the tissues and organs may not get enough oxygen. The brain is always protected in order to ensure that it receives an adequate blood supply. Compensatory mechanisms may come into effect in order to make the body lie down to protect the brain. This is where the symptom of faintness may come from as the body sends out signals that the head needs to be lowered.

Chest discomfort or pain

If the individual has pre-existing coronary heart disease and myocardial ischaemia, then an arrhythmia can provoke an angina attack.

Fatigue

If the arrhythmia is long lasting then the body expends excess energy, and a feeling of tiredness and fatigue may occur or even become the norm for the person.

Causes of arrhythmias

There are several potential causes of irregular heart rhythms:

- Coronary heart disease
- Electrolyte disturbances in the blood – as a result of dehydration or endocrine problems. The main electrolytes at play here are sodium and potassium
- Consequences and complications of a heart attack
- Post heart surgery issues
- Thyrotoxicosis – thyroid gland overactivity
- Excess alcohol
- Smoking
- Excess caffeine
- Beta blockers.

Sometimes, as a result of any of the above factors, a part of the heart other than its natural pacemaker, the sinoatrial node, will fire off a signal, which may manifest itself as a single extra beat or an abnormal rhythm.

Diagnosis

The doctor will examine the heart and feel the pulse. This may give a good idea of what the problem is, but further investigations will be necessary:

ECG

This is the first and the main test. It may show an abnormal rhythm if the heart is beating irregularly at that time. In many cases it is diagnostic.

Holter monitor

This is an ambulatory monitor that is attached to the patient while they go about their normal activities for 24–48 hours. Ambulatory means that it can be worn when walking. It will record an ECG from its chest leads, which is all that is needed to get an idea about abnormal rhythm.

An event meter

This is very similar to a Holter monitor, except it does not monitor continuously. It can be triggered by the patient themselves when they start to experience symptoms. This is of value if they only occasionally have the sensations that need to be monitored.

Echocardiogram

This may show how the heart is functioning during an arrhythmia.

Cardiac catheterisation and electrophysiological studies

This is a study of the heart carried out in a catheter lab. It is sometimes called an EP test and it is done when there are fast arrhythmias. Essentially a catheter is introduced into the heart via a vein in the groin. It will be threaded under X-ray control into a position inside the heart. An electrode at the tip can be used to stimulate and record electrical activity within the heart.

The test usually takes two to three hours. As we learnt in Chapter 11, when we talked about angiograms, the person needs to remain in hospital for a few hours after such a procedure while a doctor or nurse maintains pressure on the site of the catheter insertion in order to prevent a haematoma, a blood collection, from forming.

Sometimes the procedure will be combined with 'catheter ablation', whereby the catheter is used to deliver radiofrequency energy to ablate (destroy) some of the conducting tissue of a heart area identified as causing an arrhythmia. This may solve the problem, but it may have to be followed by the insertion of a pacemaker some weeks afterwards.

Types of arrhythmias

There are four types:

- Premature or extra beats
- Supraventricular arrhythmias
- Ventricular arrhythmias
- Bradyarrhythmias.

Premature or extra beats

These are the most common type and are usually harmless. They may not cause any symptoms at all. The individual may experience an occasional thump or fluttering in the chest or feel that they have missed a beat. Any of these can occur when the person is stressed or if they are excessively tired after exertion, or if they have had too many stimulants.

Supraventricular arrhythmias

These are tachyarrhythmias, or fast heart rates. They start above the ventricles, either in the atria or in the atrioventricular node.

There are four types:

- Atrial fibrillation
- Atrial flutter
- Paroxysmal supraventricular tachycardia
- Wolff-Parkinson-White syndrome.

Atrial fibrillation

This is common and has to be taken seriously, because it can form clots within the heart, which, in turn, may be pumped around the body and lodge in a brain artery.

The heart has four chambers. In atrial fibrillation the two upper chambers, the atria, do not beat in harmony with the rest of the heart, but quiver. As a result the overall function of the heart becomes less efficient and the heart may start to fail, the result being that the individual gets short of breath.

Because the atria do not effectively pump the blood out, the blood inside them becomes sluggish. This makes clot formation more likely. This happens more often in the left atrium, so a clot can easily be flicked out into the blood supply to the brain.

Atrial fibrillation is commonest after the age of 65 and is usually the result of some degree of atherosclerosis causing coronary heart disease. It can also occur at younger ages in people with advanced uncontrolled hypertension or hyperthyroidism (overactive thyroid), or after a heart attack. People with problems associated with the mitral valve of the heart, or with certain lung disorders, including emphysema, are also susceptible. And it may even be congenital (present from birth).

If a medical examination reveals the presence of a murmur then it should be precisely diagnosed, possibly involving a referral to a specialist.

KEY POINTS

- 2–4 per cent of people with atrial fibrillation without a history of transient ischaemic attack (mini-stroke) or major stroke *will* have a major stroke within a year.
- If they go on to have a mini-stroke, their risk increases to 20–30 per cent.
- There are 50,000 new cases of atrial fibrillation each year in the UK.
- One in 200 people aged 50–60 have atrial fibrillation.
- One in ten people over 80 have atrial fibrillation.

There are different ways of treating atrial fibrillation:

- Reduce the heart rate with drugs like beta blockers.
- Reduce the rhythm of the heart:

1. With cardioversion – this is an electric shock to jolt the heart back into a normal rhythm; or
2. With antiarrhythmic drugs, such as beta blockers, verapamil (a calcium channel blocker) or amiodarone.

- Thin the blood through either:
  1. Anticoagulation with drugs like warfarin – to prevent blood clots being formed by the butter-churn action of the fibrillating atria. This is 80 per cent likely to prevent clots; or
  2. Antiplatelet drugs like aspirin, if the patient cannot be anticoagulated. This is 20 per cent likely to prevent clots.
- Other treatments: including treatments for thyroid problems or high blood pressure, or surgery for heart valve problems.

Atrial flutter

This is similar to atrial fibrillation, but whereas in atrial fibrillation the atria beat totally irregularly, in atrial flutter they beat fast but more regularly. It is usually caused by coronary artery disease and is common after heart surgery. It may develop into atrial fibrillation.

Paroxysmal supraventricular tachycardia (PST)

This is a very rapid heart rate that starts and ends suddenly. It often occurs in young people. The electrical signals that start in the atria travel towards the ventricles and then boomerang back into the atria causing extra heartbeats. It is usually not harmful.

Wolff-Parkinson-White syndrome

This is a special type of PST. It is caused by electrical signals passing down an accessory (extra) 'bundle of His' to cause the ventricles to beat very fast. It can be dangerous.

The 'bundles of His' are the specialised conducting bundles that transmit electrical impulses from the atrioventricular node down between the ventricles to the Purkinje system (the network of specialised conducting tissues I mentioned in Chapter 1).

Destroying the accessory bundle by catheter ablation (see above) may be curative.

Ventricular arrhythmias

As their name suggests, these originate in the ventricles. They are all potentially dangerous and require emergency treatment.

Ventricular tachycardia

The ventricles beat very fast and regularly. An episode may last seconds or longer. If they only last seconds they are not too problematic, but if they last longer they can be very dangerous and transform into ventricular fibrillation.

Ventricular fibrillation

This is extremely dangerous, requiring urgent action. The ventricles quiver, as the atria do in atrial fibrillation, but if this lasts for more than a few seconds cardiac arrest is likely, because the ventricles do not have a chance to fill up and the circulation of blood is compromised. The patient is liable to be rendered unconscious and an electrical shock to the heart must be given to defibrillate it (using the special machine known, not surprisingly, as a defibrillator).

Bradyarrhythmias

These are arrhythmias with a slow heart rate of fewer than 50 beats per minute. People who are very fit may have a heart rate of fewer than 60, but this is normal for them. Bradyarrhythmias may be caused by:

- Heart attacks
- Underactive thyroid glands
- Problems with potassium blood levels
- Side effects of beta blockers, channel blockers or digoxin.

There are two main problems with bradyarrhythmias – sinus node dysfunction and heart block:

Sinus node dysfunction

This is due to an abnormally functioning sinoatrial node (as you may recall from Chapter 1, this is the natural pacemaker of the heart), and it tends to occur in the elderly (in about one in 600 people over the age of 65). It may cause the following symptoms:

- Stokes-Adams attacks – these are faints due to insufficient blood being pumped to the brain
- Dizziness
- Angina pains
- Fatigue
- Nausea
- Palpitations
- Breathlessness.

Diagnosis is by ambulatory ECG and stress exercise test, and the treatment is to have a pacemaker fitted.

Heart block

There are various degrees of heart block (which means that the electrical impulse is delayed somewhere on its way from the sinoatrial node to the ventricles). It can occur anywhere in the electrical conducting tissue, at the atrioventricular node or in the 'bundles of His'. It tends to cause an irregular heartbeat and a very slow pulse, which may be insufficient to maintain an adequate circulation.

A pacemaker is likely to be needed in the case of 'complete heart block' (the highest level of three).

BUNDLE BRANCH BLOCK

This is a pattern that is often only picked up incidentally on an ECG. If there is an interruption of the impulses down the 'bundles of His', of which there is a right and a left branch supplying the two respective ventricles, then the ventricles may beat slightly out of synch. This causes the appearance of a double-peaked, M-shaped main complex on the ECG, instead of the single peak of the QRS complex on a normal ECG reading (see Figure 18).

Right bundle branch block can be found in healthy individuals, but further investigation is necessary in order to eliminate certain conditions affecting the right side of the heart or the lungs.

Left bundle branch block is often a sign of underlying heart disease and further investigations will be performed to more accurately assess the condition.

Drugs used to treat arrhythmias

There are several types of drugs that may be used to treat the various arrhythmias, and they are classified according to which parts of the heart they work on:

Antiarrhythmic drugs

Supraventricular antiarrhythmic drugs

These work above the ventricles and include denosine, verapamil, cardiac glycosides (like digoxin) and beta blockers.

Combined supraventricular and ventricular antiarrhythmic drugs

These work on both areas of heart irregularity and include amiodarone, beta blockers, disopyramide, flecainide and propafenone.

Ventricular antiarrhythmic drugs

These only act on the ventricles and include lidocaine and moricizine.

Anticoagulants and antiplatelets

These both reduce the risk of blood clot and therefore of having a stroke.

Aspirin

Aspirin is antithrombotic. This means that it prevents the formation of a thrombus, or blood clot. It is also called an antiplatelet drug, because it stops platelets from sticking together and producing a blood clot.

Aspirin is known to have many beneficial effects. It is a painkiller, an antipyretic (lowers temperature) and an anti-inflammatory. More and more research is demonstrating that in low daily doses it reduces the risk of heart attacks, strokes and various types of cancer.

Its effectiveness in reducing heart attacks and strokes comes about because it blocks the action of an enzyme called cyclooxygenase-1, usually referred to as COX-1. This enzyme is present inside many types of cells, including the platelets, where it is responsible for releasing a chemical called thromboxane that causes platelets to clump and stick together to encourage a clot to form.

This clumping of platelets generally has a beneficial effect in the body, because it is the way that we heal wounds, but on the other hand it can be extremely dangerous when it produces a clot inside a blood vessel, such as in the development of a coronary thrombosis. Aspirin will prevent that blood clotting from happening, so it greatly reduces the risk of a coronary artery being blocked by a blood clot.

It is recommended that 300 mg of aspirin is given on admission to hospital with acute coronary syndrome. It is then generally continued as 75 mg indefinitely, as long as there are no contraindications, in order to prevent a further myocardial infarction.

It should not be given to anyone who is allergic to it, or who has previously had a haemorrhagic tendency, or who has had a dyspepsia problem upon taking it, although it may be possible in some patients with past mild dyspepsia to give a proton-pump inhibitor drug such as omeprazole at the same time in order to counter the dyspepsia problem.

The dosage of aspirin needed to prevent a second stroke is usually 75 to 150 mg.

> **ASPIRIN HAS LOTS OF POTENTIAL SIDE EFFECTS**
>
> You should *never* take aspirin if you:
>
> - Have a history of stomach ulceration.
> - Have a history of asthma.
> - Have had a haemorrhagic stroke.
> - Have any blood disorder or inherited condition, which could predispose you to bleeding.
> - Have had an allergic reaction to aspirin at any time in your life – there would then be the danger of having an anaphylactic reaction, a serious, potentially life-threatening allergic reaction characterised by low blood pressure, shock and difficulty breathing. It is a medical emergency.
> - Are under 16 years old.
> - Are on drugs like anticoagulants, or other drugs which could interact with aspirin to increase the risk of a bleed.

Anticoagulants

Generally, their role is in the treatment of underlying conditions, such as atrial fibrillation, which may predispose an individual to clot formation.

As we have already seen, warfarin has been the main oral anticoagulant up until recently, but two other oral anticoagulants, dabigatran and rivaroxaban, are also now being used in the treatment of patients with atrial fibrillation, in order to reduce their risk of stroke. The National Institute for Health and Care Excellence (NICE) recommends that the latter two should be used in patients with non-valvular atrial fibrillation, meaning atrial fibrillation in the absence of a heart valve problem. For patients with atrial fibrillation and a known heart valve problem, warfarin is still the drug of choice.

NICE also has recommendations about which patients should have aspirin and which should have an anticoagulant, based on their CHADS2 risk assessment system.

The CHADS2 algorithm is used for calculating the risk of having a stroke for patients with non-valvular atrial fibrillation. It is also used to determine whether treatment with anticoagulants or antiplatelets is needed.

- C = Congestive heart failure
- H = Hypertension
- A = Age of 75 years or over
- D = Presence of diabetes mellitus
- S2 = Prior stroke or mini-stroke, or history of thromboembolism.

One point is allotted to each of the first four parameters if they are present and two points are allotted if S2 applies. The greater the CHADS2 score, the greater the risk of stroke within the next year.

CHADS2 score	STROKE RISK %	RECOMMENDATION
0	1.9	Aspirin
1	2.8	Aspirin or anticoagulant
2	4.0	Anticoagulant
3	5.9	Anticoagulant
4	8.5	Anticoagulant
5	12.5	Anticoagulant
6	18.2	Anticoagulant

A modified version is also used with additional criteria, which gives more accurate results for lower-risk patients. But for our purposes here, CHADS2 gives the general idea.

Thus, for patients with atrial fibrillation classified at low risk of a stroke, i.e. with a CHADS2 score of zero, aspirin in a daily dose of 75 to 300 mg should be given, assuming no contraindications.

In patients with atrial fibrillation classified at moderate risk of a stroke, i.e. a CHADS2 score of 1, a daily dose of 75 to 300 mg of aspirin should be given but anticoagulation can also be considered as an alternative.

In patients with atrial fibrillation classified at high risk of a stroke, i.e. with a CHADS2 score of 2 or above, an anticoagulant should be given, provided there is no contraindication. If there is a contraindication, then aspirin should be considered, provided there are no contraindications to it.

As I have said, anticoagulants like warfarin are probably 80 per cent likely to prevent clot formation, whereas aspirin is about 20 per cent likely to prevent clots. One would have thought it is better to opt for the higher protection, but in medicine it is always a case of balancing risk against benefit. The problem with using warfarin or the other anticoagulants for everyone is that there is a significant risk of haemorrhage with them. In someone who has had a large ischaemic area of infarction, there would therefore be a risk of a haemorrhagic stroke.

CARDIOVERSION

If medical treatment has been unsuccessful in controlling persistent atrial fibrillation or ventricular tachycardia, then cardioversion may be used. This involves giving the patient a general anaesthetic and then delivering an electric shock to

> the chest wall. This shocks the heart and may re-establish a normal rhythm. Cardioversion is usually carried out as a day case procedure.
>
> It sometimes works for a period of time before atrial fibrillation recurs, and it may be possible to repeat with a further cardioversion.

Devices

There are several types of devices that can be implanted into the body to control arrhythmias.

Pacemaker

This is used to regulate bradyarrhythmias, such as 'complete heart block'. A small box containing a pulse generator is implanted under the skin near the collarbone. An insulated wire extends from the box to the heart where it is tethered.

The older pacemakers had fixed rates, whereas the newer ones are highly sophisticated and contain microcomputers which turn on when needed and off when the heart is beating well. In other words, they pace on demand. Most pacemakers last for 7–15 years and then need to be changed. They are checked regularly at pacemaker clinics and can be reprogrammed externally.

Implantable cardioverter defibrillator (ICD)

This is a device used to treat ventricular tachycardia and ventricular fibrillation. These are both life-threatening conditions and this device is therefore a life-saving one.

An electronic box is implanted under the skin, as with a pacemaker. It continually monitors the heart rhythm and if it detects an arrhythmia it can deliver electrical impulses in different ways in order to re-establish normal rhythm. It can deliver the following:

Antitachycardia pacing

If the heart is beating too fast, the ICD emits a series of small impulses to override the tachycardia and slow the heart down to a normal rhythm.

Cardioversion

If the chambers of the heart are beating out of synch, the ICD can emit a low-energy shock to jolt it back into a synchronised rhythm.

Defibrillation

If the heart is beating very fast or very irregularly, as it does in ventricular fibrillation, there will be a danger of cardiac arrest. The ICD will in those circumstances deliver a high-energy shock in order to defibrillate and restore a normal rhythm.

Antibradycardic pacing

The ICD may also have a pacing ability if it detects a very slow heart rate.

Chapter 15

After a heart attack

Life after a heart attack can be very different. The fact that an event of such enormity has occurred inevitably makes one reassess one's life. Any heart attack is potentially fatal, so it is normal to feel frightened. But after the event has passed and you are out of danger, there is relief. Then there will be other concerns.

Cardiac rehabilitation

After a heart attack, and once any irregularity has been stabilised and any treatment needed for heart failure is under way, it is usual to begin a period known as cardiac rehabilitation.

The programme of rehabilitation starts in hospital and continues for several weeks on an outpatient basis. The aims of this programme are to give advice about how to make the best recovery, and how to adopt lifestyle changes that will maintain health and reduce the risk of having another attack. Usually a nurse will run through all of these things, advising on what you should and shouldn't do once you leave hospital.

Rehabilitation continues with sessions at the hospital a few weeks after the heart attack. This is when it is safe to start exercising. A physiotherapist or specialist nurse will run a session, where you will meet other people who are going through the same programme. Some will have very recently had a heart attack, like you. Others will be further on.

An exercise schedule will be tailored to your health and fitness. Some people may not have exercised for years and they need to gradually get used to more activity.

Generally a session will last for about an hour, twice a week, for six to eight weeks. Relaxation techniques may be shown, and there will be further advice about lifestyle and advice about how to make changes. Other professionals, like doctors and pharmacists, may be in attendance or be called upon to give advice.

The main lifestyle changes to reduce the risk of having a further attack are as follows:

- Stop smoking.
- Lose excess weight.
- Carry out regular physical activity – the recommended amount for adults is 30 minutes on at least five days a week.
- Eat a low-fat and high-fibre diet with at least five portions of fruit and vegetables a day and two portions of fish (one oily) a week.
- Do not drink more than four units of alcohol a day for men or three units a day for women.

> **STOP SMOKING**
>
> NHS stop-smoking services offer support that works. You are up to four times more likely to quit smoking successfully if you go to your local NHS stop-smoking service and use stop-smoking medicines, than if you try to quit using willpower alone. They can help you with:
>
> - Strategies
> - Chewing gum
> - Nicotine patches
> - Drugs – e.g. bupropion (Zyban) or varenicline (Champix)
> - NHS Direct helpline advice.

Work

The area of the heart muscle that was damaged will take a few weeks to recover. That is why exercise is not advised until about two weeks after a heart attack. This should be gentle to begin with, gradually increasing over the six to eight weeks of the cardiac rehabilitation programme. The aim is to get back to normality in two to three months.

If your job is of a sedentary type then it is reasonable to get back to work by eight weeks. If it is of a more strenuous type then three months would be reasonable.

Driving

This is an important question for most people.

Car or motorcycle licence

You don't need to tell the DVLA. However, you should stop driving for at least a month after your heart attack and only start driving again when your doctor tells you that you are safe to do so.

Bus, coach or lorry licence

Holders of special licenses must tell the DVLA they have had heart problems by filling in form VOCH1. The form is downloadable from the DVLA website and the return address is on the form.

Sex life

This is an important area of life and most people should be able to get back to a full and normal sex life within a few weeks. Generally, it is advised to wait about three weeks, but many people do not find that their libido returns that quickly, and so it is sensible to be open and candid with your partner and avoid feeling a pressure to have sex before you are ready.

It is probably a good thing to be gentle in lovemaking during the first few weeks. Obviously, if chest pain occurs during it, then it should be discontinued. There is a possibility that it could be angina and a further medical check would be sensible. The vast majority of people, however, have no such problem.

If depression occurs, that can affect the libido, but once the depression is diagnosed and treated the libido may well improve.

Emotional recovery

After a heart attack it is normal to feel emotional. It is a potentially life-threatening event and the realisation that they could have died inevitably makes people aware of how important their heart is.

Irritability

This is common following a heart attack for several weeks and the individual may be aware that they are irritated by things that would not have bothered them before. Their partner or family may feel that they have to be careful lest they provoke an outburst of anger. Talking about how you feel is to be encouraged, since the old adage about a problem shared being a problem halved is very true. The mere fact that you can talk about your feelings often helps to get things into proportion.

Anxiety

This is also common, since most people will worry that they could have another attack. However, if tests have been carried out, including an angiogram, and perhaps if a stent has been put in, the individual should try to focus on the positives. That is, they should bear in mind that their coronary artery blood flow has been improved and that they are in a better position in terms of having another attack than they were before the first one.

Most people will gradually feel better and become less anxious as time passes and they experience a sense of returning to normal life, and possibly also a return to work if appropriate.

Depression

Feeling a bit down in the dumps following a heart attack is also common (about 20 per cent of people will suffer from depression after a heart attack), but the feeling does tend to go as the individual starts to physically feel better and less tired.

The reasons for the depression can relate to fear of death and/or fear about the future. Or they can be caused by anxiety about the rest of the family. Talking about it will usually help.

Depression may make the individual feel weepy. They may notice that they are worse in the morning and tend to get less depressed as the day goes on. Apathy is common, so the individual may need encouragement to do things and aim for a return to normal life. They may lose their appetite and they may complain that there is simply no point in their treatment or in them going on living. These are all indicative of a marked depression.

The important thing is not to bottle the feelings up. There are generally four conditions that are strong indications that you need help and you should seek it from your doctor. These are:

- If your feelings of depression are persisting and not getting better, or if they are getting worse.

- If your depressed mood is affecting your life, whether in relation to family, social life, work or leisure.

- If you start having morbid thoughts and feel useless and of no value.

- If you contemplate or cannot stop thinking about self-harming or suicide.

Positive support is what is needed and many people will respond to this after a few days. For those who do not begin to feel better, it may be necessary for them to have a course of antidepressants. The choice of antidepressant will be decided by relevant medical staff. It is likely that the course will need to be taken for several weeks and more often than not several months, after which it can usually be stopped. They usually do not start working for about a week to two weeks.

The life cycle

The emotional reaction to having a cardiovascular event like a heart attack or a stroke can be very severe. In my own practice I devised a simple model that I call the 'life cycle' to try to help with emotional problems and/or chronic physical symptoms. It is not rocket science, but it can give the individual a framework and a means of helping him or herself. We shall return to this in Chapter 17.

Chapter 16

Managing hypertension

As we saw in Chapter 4, hypertension puts the person at risk of several problems, so its control is of paramount importance. It tends not to cause any symptoms, so you will not know that you have a problem with it until you have your blood pressure taken.

It is sensible for adults to have their blood pressure checked at least every five years until the age of 80. It should be done annually after that. If it is found to be borderline, your doctor will want to monitor it more frequently.

Diagnosis of blood pressure

Your doctor or the practice nurse will measure your blood pressure using a regularly maintained machine. Practices have all of their sphygmomanometers calibrated, so that all practitioners and nurses are measuring blood pressure with the same accuracy.

The blood pressure is usually taken when you are seated. A blood pressure cuff is wrapped around the upper arm and is then inflated. It will either be done with an automated digital machine or by using an aneroid (mechanical with a needle dial) sphygmomanometer and a stethoscope. If the latter is used, then the examiner listens to the Korotkoff sounds that were mentioned in Chapter 4.

As we have seen, the blood pressure is recorded as two figures, the upper being the systolic blood pressure, the pressure attained as the heart beats, and the lower being the diastolic pressure, which represents the pressure in the circulation as the heart relaxes between beats.

A reading of 140/90 mmHG is already suspect (i.e. too high) and requires further monitoring (see box below for information about grades of hypertension). In the past, three readings on different days were taken and the average worked out, but now ambulatory blood pressure monitoring (AMBP) will probably be offered if the pressure seems abnormal, since this is regarded as a more accurate means of doing it (and several studies have shown this to be the case).[17]

As we saw in Chapter 14, the AMBP involves wearing a cuff attached to a monitor. It is not intrusive and allows the person to go about their daily business. Blood pressure readings are taken every 20 minutes during the day and every hour overnight.

This has the advantage of overcoming any 'white coat syndrome', the phenomenon that some people's blood pressure goes up when they see a health practitioner.

Not all practices have the ambulatory facility, but it is also possible to do home blood-pressure monitoring (HBPM) using an automated machine provided for the purpose. The individual takes two readings twice a day, in the morning and evening, i.e. four in total each day. Those readings are then averaged out.

> The National Institute for Health and Care Excellence (NICE) recommends the following definitions for the three perceived grades of hypertension:
>
> - Stage 1 – BP in surgery is equal to or above 140/90 mmHg and subsequent ABPM or HBPM is equal to or greater than 135/85 mmHg.
> - Stage 2 – BP in surgery is equal to or greater than 160/100 mmHg and subsequent ABPM or HBPM is equal to or greater than 150/95 mmHg.
> - Severe – BP in surgery is equal to or greater than 180/110 mmHg.

People with borderline blood pressure, that is in the range 130–139/85–89 should be advised to have annual check-ups.

Special considerations

There are three additional situations that may have to be considered:

Malignant hypertension

This is exceedingly high blood pressure with a systolic of greater than 200 and/or a diastolic of greater than 130. It is accompanied by significant end organ damage (damage to major organs), such as papilloedema (swelling of the optic discs in the eyes) and possibly by a dulling of consciousness, along with inflammation of the brain or kidneys. It requires immediate investigation and treatment.

Phaeochromocytoma

This is a tumour of the adrenal gland and it produces paroxysmal hypertension, i.e. blood pressure that is raised on occasions. It may cause headaches, pallor and profuse sweating. If suspected it should be investigated immediately.

Systolic or diastolic hypertension

It is possible to have elevation of only one of the figures. It used to be considered that the diastolic was more important but studies such as the Framingham one in Massachusetts have shown that this is not the case and that systolic elevation is more likely to increase the risk of cardiovascular disease.[18]

Investigations

Most cases of hypertension are managed in general practice and only those that are perhaps due to a secondary cause, or those which have not been able to be controlled by drugs, need to be referred for specialist help. Young patients under the age of 40 are likely to be referred.

The baseline investigations needed are as follows:

- *ECG* – to assess whether the left ventricle has become enlarged due to having to pump blood through smaller blood vessels. This will show up as left ventricular hypertrophy (LVH) on the ECG.

- *Urine testing* – this is done by dipstick, to test for protein and blood in the urine. This test could indicate any possible kidney problems.

- *Blood tests* – to assess the levels of serum creatinine, urea and electrolytes, and to assess the eGFR (estimated glomerular filtration rate). These all might give indications of kidney problems.

- *Lipid profile* – to look for abnormalities in the serum cholesterol and triglyceride levels and to check the cholesterol:HDL ratio (see Chapter 10 for a reminder on lipid profiling).

- *Blood glucose level* – to test for diabetes.

In younger patients further tests may be requested, possibly prior to referral. Such further investigations may include:

- *Echocardiogram* – to assess the functioning of the heart.

- *Chest X-ray* – to assess the size of the heart.

- *Ultrasound* – to check on the kidneys.

Hospital investigations may include:

- *Renal arteriogram* – to assess the blood supply to the kidneys. Renal artery stenosis, a blockage in the main artery to the kidney, is one of the causes of secondary hypertension.

- *Endocrinological testing* – to check for various endocrine causes of hypertension (see Chapter 4).

Management of blood pressure

Not everyone with raised blood pressure will need drug treatment. Indeed, blood pressure is only one risk factor for cardiovascular disease. If it is the only risk factor that a person has, and they only have borderline blood pressure, then they may simply need regular monitoring. For those at greater risk, blood pressure can be managed in a number of different ways:

Lifestyle alteration

Attention will be given to altering lifestyle habits that may be hazardous to health. Essentially, these are all of the factors that we considered in Chapter 10. They are all relevant to blood pressure control.

To recap, the important risk factors are:

- Smoking
- Obesity
- Lack of exercise
- Excess alcohol
- Bad cholesterol levels
- High salt intake.

Drug treatment

This will be started in patients with grade 1 hypertension if there is evidence of end organ damage, e.g. changes in the retina of the eye, or indication of kidney damage. All patients with grade 2 and severe hypertension should be started on drug treatment.

As we saw in Chapter 13, there are four main groups of drugs used in the treatment of hypertension. These are:

- ACE inhibitors

- ARBs
- Calcium channel blockers
- Diuretics.

You may want to refer back to Chapter 13 for more details about these types of drugs, but here is a quick recap:

ACE inhibitors

As we have seen, these are angiotensin-converting enzyme (ACE) inhibitors. They work by dilating the blood vessels to reduce blood pressure and enhance blood flow.

ARBs

ARBs (angiotensin receptor blockers) work in a similar way to ACE inhibitors by widening blood vessels and reducing blood pressure. They may be prescribed instead of ACE inhibitors because they do not usually cause a cough.

Calcium channel blockers

These block the flow of calcium into muscle cells on the blood vessel walls, which has the effect of keeping the arterioles dilated.

Diuretics

These are water pills that make you pass more urine. They have been used in the treatment of hypertension for over 50 years, but are now considered third-line drugs.

Figure 20: The sites of action of antihypertensive drugs

Sympathetic nervous system
Beta blockers
Alpha blockers

Heart
Beta blockers

Blood vessels
Alpha blockers
Calcium channel blockers
Vasodilators
ACE inhibitors
ARBs

Kidneys
Diuretics
Beta blockers
ACE inhibitors
ARBs

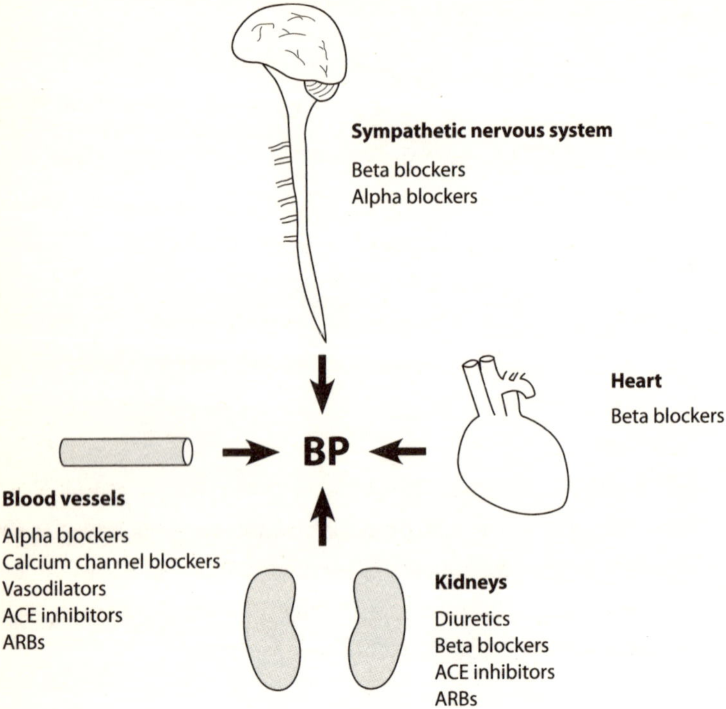

About half the people treated with these antihypertensive drugs need two or three different types. If one or more of the drugs are not tolerated by an individual, or if they are failing to adequately control blood pressure, beta blockers (see Chapters 11 and 13) or alpha blockers may be added into the equation. Alpha blockers work by relaxing your blood vessels, making it much easier for blood to flow through them, but are not usually recommended as a choice for lowering high blood pressure unless other treatments have not worked.

Chapter 17

The life cycle

We have covered a lot of ground in this book and I appreciate that it can be difficult for individuals experiencing problems after they have developed a condition to know where to start in order to help themselves. In my own practice I use a model that I call the 'life cycle' to help patients examine their life and devise strategies that they can use for self-help purposes. I do not pretend that this is any kind of rocket science. It is simply a model that many people find useful in gaining a bit of focus.

The life cycle – a summary

This term 'life cycle' may take you back to your days of studying biology, when you looked at the different life cycles of insects, fish, frogs and other creatures on the evolutionary ladder. I am not, however, using the term here in the same sense. I am using it as a model for a person's life. This has nothing to do with their development with age, but has to do instead with the different levels or spheres that make up one's life at any point in time. And you will see that there is a cycle involved in the manner in which virtually any chronic medical condition (whether physical or psychological) can affect people.

Yet to use the biology analogy a little longer, you will learn a certain amount about fish by dissecting them to look at their internal organs. But you won't know how they move and feed without studying them in water. And you won't learn about their behaviour with other fish and predators unless you observe them in a realistic environment. Even then you will not get to know about them fully unless you specialise in observing them.

So it is in medicine. In order to help someone you need to know as much as possible about their condition, their symptoms and the things that make their symptoms better or worse. And ideally you want to know about their habits, their diet, their desires, their fears, their relationships and so on. That might seem like a tall order, but if you can build up such a picture of a patient, you can see how a condition is truly affecting them throughout all levels of their life.

And building up such a picture is what you need to do in order to help yourself manage a condition in the most effective way that you can. The model enables you to build a picture of your life including the ways that the different spheres of your life interact.

There are five life spheres that we need to consider:

- *Body* – the symptoms you have, e.g. pain, stiffness, tiredness.

- *Emotion* – how you feel, e.g. anxious, sad, depressed, angry or jealous of others.

- *Mind* – the type of thoughts you have, e.g. pessimistic, negative, self-defeating.

- *Behaviour* – how you behave and interact, e.g. do you join in or do you isolate yourself by avoiding things or people? Are you developing bad habits, e.g. smoking, drinking excessively, or becoming inactive.

- *Lifestyle* – how it affects your ability to do things, your relationships, and also how events in your life impact on you.

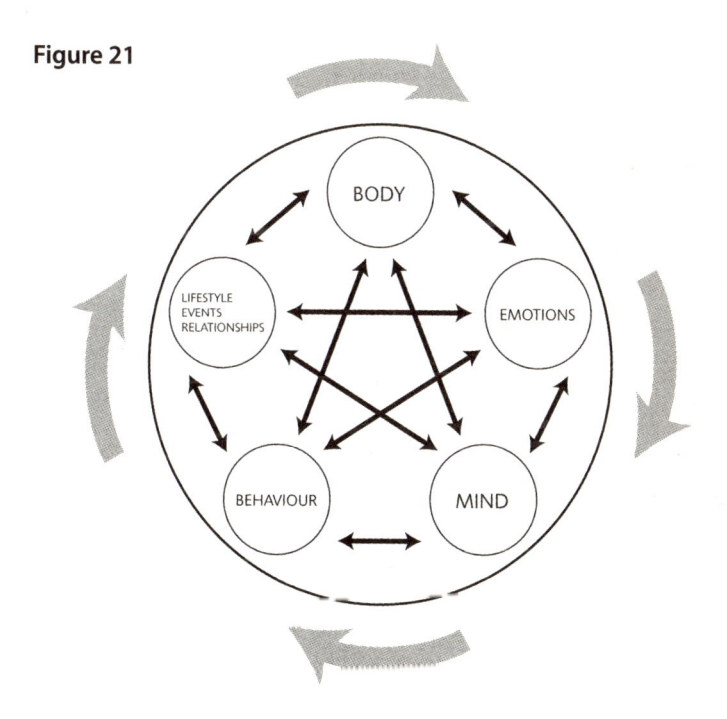

Figure 21

Now take a look at Figure 21. You will see the five spheres starting with the body sphere at the top. If you follow the figure clockwise you will see that it follows the order above – body, emotions, mind, behaviour and lifestyle. And note the outer circle that encloses the whole structure. This represents the individual's whole self, their life. In other words, the five spheres all make up part of the individual's experience of life.

Note that the outer arrows of the diagram represent a general progression, a 'life cycle', because the order represents the way that a physical condition will tend to impact on a person's life. To begin with, physical symptoms make the individual aware that something is wrong in the body. This can induce an emotional response, which could be anxiety, anger, resentment or fear. That emotion then alters the way you think, which in turn may cause you take a particular action, perhaps to reach for a drink or take a tablet. Your actions may then affect your lifestyle, stopping you from doing certain things, which in turn may affect relationships and work. And all of that can set the cycle off again.

Notice also that inside the outer ring of arrows there are double-headed arrows between the spheres. These show that every sphere impacts on every single other one. In other words, a pain, for example, impacts on all spheres of your life. On the other hand, the inner arrows give you the opportunity to use any of the other spheres to reduce the pain or to deal with it better. And with a symptom like depression, you can do exactly the same thing. It is felt in the emotional sphere, which makes you think in a particular way, which makes you then act in a particular way, which will in turn impact on your lifestyle. You may or may not feel physical symptoms but there are nonetheless lots of potential ways in any one sphere in which you can positively affect the state of depression. Just by realising this you may be able to reduce the feeling of hopelessness that tends to go hand in hand with depression, and you may start to see that you are not helpless, that there are all those potential strategies that can help you.

Use the life cycle to sketch out your life

This can be a useful thing to do. Get a notebook and make it your life cycle diary. Draw the five spheres and label them. Draw all of the arrows as in the diagram. Do it deliberately, carefully, because you are crafting something here. It is your life cycle and it deserves to look its best! Take a pride in it. Realise also that it is a dynamic thing that you are going to be able to change. Indeed, as you fill up the notebook, which you should do gradually, on a weekly basis, you will very visibly see those changes.

So, after the page with the life cycle on it, allocate two facing pages to each sphere. Make an entry on each one. For example, with the body sphere, just jot down any physical feelings that you have. It may be 'fatigue', or 'palpitations' or 'sore throat'. Whatever you are aware of. With emotions, it may be 'relief' or 'depression' that you first think of. But write words or notes that describe it better than that. What exactly are you feeling? What thoughts are you having? And so on to complete the cycle.

You will soon see that some sort of a pattern manifests itself to you. You may feel that it would work better if you were to score every entry, that is, give them a positive or a negative score. That way you can produce a number for each sphere. The emotion sphere and/or the mind sphere may initially have negative scores, but that's fine.

Some of you might prefer something more visual. You may, for example, prefer to use the cycle itself on which to enter your notes.

If needs be, you can make some spheres larger than others. The emotion and mind spheres may initially be larger than the others, but over the weeks you will hopefully be able to calibrate all five spheres as equals, not dominated by the emotions.

By focusing on certain spheres you should find that you are able to influence others and, as a result of this, you may start to find yourself on a more even keel.

Let us look more closely now at the individual spheres.

The sphere of emotion

People who are depressed will have had other people tell them to cheer up, or possibly even to pull their socks up. They may have tried telling themselves the same things. They may have gone through a sort of balance sheet in their heads, ticking off all the positives in their life in an attempt to realise that they have no need to feel down. Yet it doesn't seem to help. You can't just cheer up. You can't just tell depression to go. Something has to happen to make it go.

Let me give you an analogy. If you are feeling nervous and fearful, with butterflies in your stomach and a rapid heartbeat, you can't say 'heart, slow down' or 'tummy, settle down'. The reason is that these are physiological changes and you can't alter them by just giving an order. You have to induce a reaction that will result in them being settled, and the reaction that you need to use is a relaxation response.

There is a technique called progressive muscle relaxation, which is actually very good at producing this relaxation response. I will describe it when I come to the body sphere. It is a useful technique that many people with anxiety and depression find helpful, and it is a good example of the way that one sphere can affect another – if it can make one sphere feel more relaxed, that will automatically affect the other spheres as well.

Of course, the notes you make in your emotion sphere may not simply have the word 'depression' in it. There may be other emotions in there, like guilt, hate, irritability or hopelessness. Sometimes you need to focus on individual key features like those in order to reduce the overall weight of the emotion sphere.

Anger can affect the heart

There have been several studies linking anger with an increased risk of heart disease. An interesting piece of research from Yale University in the USA suggests that anger may have a direct effect on the heart, possibly even to the extent that it could cause irregularities of the heart, and it must therefore be possible that these could prove fatal.

You will have seen the scenario played out on television and in film many times before. Some sudden event causes a rush of emotion and a character clutches their chest and dies. It is not a piece of fiction. Many people may be aware of instances when someone has died upon receiving a shock, or when they are in the surge of a temper attack.

The Yale research looked at a group of 62 people who all had implanted defibrillators. Over a three-year period 16 per cent of the group experienced a heart irregularity that set off their implanted defibrillator while going through a mental stress test, basically involving the recall of a recent situation that had angered them.

They were all found to have the 'T-wave alternans' (also known as the 'TWA phenomenon'), which is a curious feature that some people are found to have on a stress ECG test. Effectively, when you look at an ECG tracing, the last bump in the cardiac cycle is called the T-wave. People with TWA show an alternating height pattern in that T-wave, but it is not usually apparent unless they have had a physical stress test to get the heart beating quickly. This is because the change normally is not of great amplitude. Its significance lies in the fact that it may indicate those individuals who are at risk of developing a heart irregularity.

This study is important, since it suggests that anger can provoke the same phenomenon as can a physical stress. Thus, anger seems to have a direct effect on the heart, not through causing the blood pressure to rise, but through an effect on the electrical activity of the heart.

A lot more research needs to be done on this, but it does join the body of evidence that is accumulating about the effects of anger. If you are an angry type, then it makes sense to try modifying your behaviour. By being the sort of person who explodes with rage, who fires from the hip, you may be putting your health at risk.

It is not always easy to fight an emotion, but try to develop an awareness of when you are losing your temper. Then stop and think of the consequences of firing off. Consider the options and make a careful decision. You may help your health (and others may find you more pleasant to live with).

The sphere of the mind

This is obviously the most important sphere, yet it is not the only one to focus on. I firmly believe that you need to consider all of the spheres and get them working for you. Yet the way that you think is of huge relevance because:

- Thoughts arise from emotions.
- Emotions arise from thought patterns.
- Thoughts and emotions affect and are affected by the other life spheres.

Thoughts arise from emotions

The sort of thoughts that you have are in part determined by the emotions that you are feeling. If you wake up in the morning and you feel happy, then the train of thought that you have is liable to go in a different direction from the train that you will have if you wake up feeling fearful, guilty, angry or sad.

Emotions do not of course just turn off if you tell them to change. You have to make them change, and one of the most effective ways to do this is by thinking positively.

It is not always that easy, I admit, and the person who is depressed is probably trying to do it all the time often without succeeding. People who are depressed, or who have experienced depression, often talk about the constant battle or struggle with their mood. The problem can often be that negative thinking reinforces negative emotion.

Emotions arise from thought patterns

This is extremely important to understand. People who experience depression do not think in the same way as people who never get depressed. They seem to have depressive thinking, which means they find it difficult to think positively.

Dr Aaron Beck, one of the originators of cognitive therapy, observed that depressive thinking comes about because of what he called the cognitive triad, the tendency that depression-prone people have to view themselves, the world and the future in a negative manner:

- *Personal view* – they have a poor image of themselves as individuals, because they feel unworthy and inadequate, and that they have to make excuses for themselves.

- *World view* – they can only see the negative side of things, especially in relation to themselves. They will only see what they have done wrong, not what they did well, and they will take criticism to heart.

- *Future view* – this tends to be bleak and gloomy. In part this relates to their feeling of personal inadequacy and the sense that everything that can go wrong will go wrong and possibly even be perceived as their fault.

These views are not always conscious, which is why the life cycle diary might just help some depressed people to break out of Dr Beck's cognitive triad.

Thoughts and emotions affect and are affected by the other life spheres

This is also fundamental. If you are feeling sad and depressed and it is making you feel worthless and unattractive, the inevitable consequence is to withdraw and isolate yourself from situations where that feeling might be overwhelming. In other words, the emotion induces and reinforces the thought that you are less than worthy. The behaviour you adopt is to hide away and withdraw.

But you could try something different in order to tackle that fear of exposing yourself. You could adopt a different habit, perhaps try running (behaviour and body spheres), or join a club, or meet relatives and friends more often (lifestyle sphere).

Cultivate optimism

See if you can reap the benefits of positive thinking. Instead of thinking 'I can't do it because I've never done it before', try thinking 'it's an opportunity to learn'. Or instead of 'there is no way this will work for me', try 'let me see if I can make this work'. Do not accept the false belief that because something bad happened once, it will happen again. Start looking on the bright side and expect good things to occur.

Cultivate mindfulness

Mindfulness-based cognitive therapy and mindfulness-based stress reduction are well-understood practices that are often advocated as an eight-week course in order to help people between depression episodes to stay well. It seems to be successful in reducing relapses by 50 per cent.

Mindfulness is a Buddhist practice that involves paying attention to the present moment, deliberately, without judgment. It is a means of experiencing the moment without being sucked into thinking of how the moment is affecting you or your future. It is simply being. People who are depressed cannot readily do this, because they worry constantly about the before and after of their feelings and actions.

For example, pick any activity of normal life, such as drinking a cup of tea or coffee. If you are depressed, the act of drinking the tea or coffee will probably give little pleasure, since your mind will not be involved in the act of drinking, but will be off somewhere else following a train of thought that is reinforcing a negative emotion. Mindfulness would allow you to focus on the cup of tea or coffee, the way that it was produced, the taste, the smell, the temperature, the feeling that drinking it induces.

So cultivating mindfulness, focusing on a particular activity rather than allowing the mind to wonder into fruitless negativity, is a key strategy for many people in overcoming stress or depression, and it can be applied to many different situations at any time of the day. When driving, for example, rather than allowing the mind to wander to other matters, which it does with most people, focus on the skill of driving. Regrasp the pleasure that you obtained when you first learnt to drive. Focus on the comfort of the seat, the pleasantness of the world around you. What you are really doing is disengaging the autopilot that can lead to boredom or depression.

The sphere of behaviour

This is all to do with the actions, habits and things that you do. Depressive thinking so often leads to depressive actions, which reinforce feelings of poor self-esteem. So, when you feel down, don't habitually reach for the cigarettes, the glass of wine or the bottle of beer. Don't order a helping of junk food. Instead, try to think of something to do that is completely out of the norm for you.

Changing habitat helps to change habits. Think of a place where you permit yourself to lapse into depressive habits then change the habitat – perhaps designate the usual room to be the place where it will no longer be appropriate to smoke or drink. Or instead of going outside with a packet of cigarettes, change the habitat to the kitchen and make a loaf of bread. Stay inside in the warmth and revel in the fact that you no longer smell of stale tobacco.

So change the things that you do and focus on the new things in a mindful way, enjoying the moment, disengaging the autopilot that allows you to punish yourself with negative thinking. Instead of allowing yourself to feel depressed, think positively, do things positively and focus on the joy of the moment. Little by little, piece by piece, you will change that negative feeling or habit.

The sphere of lifestyle

Friends, family, work; they all have their plusses and minuses. In depression, the minuses are what you see. Yet with mindfulness and optimistic thinking, you can change all that. Revel in the family. Enjoy being with friends. Take up new activities. Learn a language, take up yoga or meditation, start writing poetry or a novel.

Do different things to get yourself out of the rut, however comfortable that rut may seem to be.

The sphere of body

This is about body awareness. Be aware of the positive attributes of the body. Even if you are aware of physical symptoms or if you suffer a physical condition, there are still things about your body that you can enjoy. You need to be comfortable in your own skin. You need to enjoy being you.

If you feel less fit than you think you should be, then do some exercise. This is always good for you, and we will look at the options and benefits in the final chapter.

Progressive muscle relaxation

This is a technique that is often used in hypnotherapy in order to deepen a state of relaxation. There is no great mystery about it and I recommend it to you as a relaxation means.

Sit back in an easy chair or lie down somewhere you will not be disturbed by a telephone or any other interruption. Take your shoes off. Close your eyes and just tell yourself that you are going to relax all of your muscles. Tell yourself that as your muscles relax they will become less uncomfortable (use the word 'uncomfortable' rather than 'painful').

Now clench your fists tightly for a count of seven. As you do this focus your attention on the tightness in the hands, feeling it increase as you count to seven. Then suddenly let it go, and tell yourself that instead of tension there is now increasing relaxation in those muscles of the hand. And tell yourself that they will get even more relaxed as you count to 15.

Now clench your fists and this time also tense the muscles of your feet by trying to clench the toes. Do this for a count of seven, exactly as before. Then release the tension suddenly and let the relaxation deepen for a count of 15.

Now clench all of the muscles of your arms and legs, in exactly the same way. Tense for seven and relax for 15.

Then tense all of your limb muscles and clench your buttocks together, at the same time tensing your stomach and neck and face muscles. Screw your eyes tightly closed as you count to seven, and then release suddenly and relax for 15.

Then tell yourself that your muscles are now going to relax totally and that they will continue to relax and feel more comfortable when you stop. Now imagine that a wave of relaxation is moving all the way up over your body from your feet, up your legs, up your back and chest to your neck. Let that same feeling pass through both arms and up through your neck to your head, relaxing all of the muscles as it moves up to the top of your head and back down over your face.

Tell yourself that you will just enjoy that feeling for a minute or so and if you fall asleep, all well and good. But after the time is up, tell yourself that your muscles feel good and will continue to feel better and better each time that you do this.

It is as simple as that. And the thing is, the muscles will get less uncomfortable. Just make it something that you do every day.

Putting it all together

I said that this was not rocket science, yet it is a practical model that people do find useful to at least begin to address their problems and stay well. Get a notebook, do the exercises that I mentioned, practice mindfulness, start to become an optimist, and change habits and habitats.

The model is not intended as a sort of substitute for conventional care. It is simply a means of looking at the different spheres of your life to see how you can introduce self-help. It can also be used to see how any therapies and medications that have been prescribed might dovetail with the other areas of your life.

KEY POINTS

- Be aware of the cognitive triad of depressive thinking – personal view, world view, future view. You can change them.
- Mindfulness is the way to focus on the moment, and seek pleasure and joy in everyday activities.
- Optimists enjoy life; pessimists are more liable to depression. Be an optimist.
- Working on the other spheres of your life cycle can have a positive knock-on effect to your sphere of emotion.

Chapter 18

A healthy diet and taking some exercise

Diet

Getting your diet right can certainly reduce your risk of further heart trouble, but what do we mean by diet? To many people the word 'diet' implies a food restriction regime in order to lose weight. That is actually a slimming diet. The word diet simply means the food that you take in. Starting with a look at the Mediterranean diet, I am going to focus on the positive effects of anti-inflammatory foods, because the inflammation found in junk food seems to be one of the factors that predisposes to atherosclerosis and therefore coronary artery disease.

The Mediterranean diet

It is always difficult to try to determine which factors are hazardous to health and which are beneficial. A landmark piece of research was done in the 1950s and 1960s by Professor Ancel Keys at the University of Minnesota in the USA. This was called the Seven Countries Study. In this research, he and an international team of scientists studied the health of over 12,000 men from seven countries: the USA, Japan, Italy, Finland, Greece, the Netherlands and Yugoslavia. When all the research was analysed, a clear and predictable pattern emerged. In the Mediterranean and Asian regions of the world (Greece, Japan and southern Italy) where vegetables, grains, fruits, beans and fish formed a major part of the diet, heart disease was found to be rare. By contrast, in those countries where people consumed a lot of red meat, cheese and other foods high in saturated fat, such as in the USA and Finland, the rates of heart disease were found to be very high.

Since then there have been numerous studies that have repeatedly found the so-called Mediterranean diet to be associated with better health. Portugal, of course, is not on the Mediterranean coast, yet it is the European country with the most typical of what we think of as a Mediterranean diet. Essentially, such a diet is rich in olive oil, grains, fruits, nuts, vegetables and fish, and includes a moderate amount of wine, but is low in meat, dairy products and other alcohol.

A report just published from Italy, which followed over a million people for up to 18 years showed that people who eat a strict Mediterranean diet are at less risk of developing heart disease, cancer, Parkinson's disease and Alzheimer's disease. This is very important, since it suggests that many chronic conditions can be reduced simply by eating a particular type of diet. At the heart of this diet is fish, which really is so good for you.

The characteristics of the Mediterranean diet in slightly more detail are as follows:

- High levels of fruits and vegetables, breads and other cereals, potatoes, beans, nuts and seeds.

- Olive oil is the only fat allowed.

- Moderate amounts of dairy products, fish and poultry, but very little red meat.

- Eggs are allowed, but no more than four per week and no more than one on any day.

- Wine is consumed in moderate amounts – two glasses per day for men, one glass for women.

The fish and the olive oil seem to be two of the most significant features of the diet. Olive oil is rich in monounsaturated fatty acids, and it has been suggested that its benefit may be in improving the way that serotonin, the 'happiness neurotransmitter', is bound to its receptors. Oily fish is rich in omega-3 essential fatty acids, which are said to have an anti-inflammatory effect.

OILY FISH IS SO GOOD FOR YOU

The Portuguese consume more fish than any other country in Europe, and it is thought that this is reflected in their very low incidence of heart disease. In the league table of deaths from heart attacks, Slovakia has the worst rate, with 216 deaths per 100,000 of the population. The UK has 122, while Portugal has 56. Only Spain, France and Japan are lower.

A short lesson about fats and oils

Everyone knows that you must not take too much fat into your system, and we hear much about the benefits of various types of oils. Understandably, there is a lot of confusion about fats and oils, so I shall try to present my own understanding as simply as possible.

There are three basic types of fats – saturated, monounsaturated and polyunsaturated:

Saturated fats

These are found in animal products such as meat, eggs, and dairy products. In general, these are considered 'bad' fats, since they have a tendency to push up your cholesterol and promote inflammation. They do this because arachidonic acid, one of the fatty acids found in these fats, is broken down by enzymes into prostaglandins and leukotrienes, both of which are known to trigger inflammation.

Monounsaturated fats

These are found in various nuts (including peanuts, walnuts and almonds), avocados and olive oil. They help to lower cholesterol and they are 'good' fats, which means they can help to reduce inflammation.

Polyunsaturated fats

These are the best ones, and they are found in seafood and fish, corn oil and sunflower oil. They help to lower cholesterol and they are also anti-inflammatory. They are composed of two groups of essential fatty acids, called omega-3 and omega- 6. In general, omega-3s have more anti-inflammatory effect than omega-6s, and the Mediterranean diet has a better balance between the two types than the British diet.

There are two types of omega-3s, those with long chains and those with short chains. The long chains are mainly found in oily fish. The two main ones are called eicosapentaenoic acid (EPA) and docosahexaenoic acid (DHA). These are anti-inflammatory and they have been found to be good for both arthritis and the heart, and, seemingly, also depression.

Short-chain omega-3s are found in foods like soya, flax, pumpkin seeds, walnuts and leafy green vegetables. They can be converted by the body into the long-chain fatty acids that do the most good.

You will find that lots of foods, like spreads, juices and even milk have added omega-3s. This is good in that the average British diet is really quite deficient in omega-3s. Yet the thing is that it is more efficient to get the omega-3s in their natural form, i.e. from oily fish such as salmon, mackerel and sardines. Aim at having two, or even better, three portions a week.

But take care if you are prone to gout! This is not because of the omega oils, but because of the high purine content of oily fish. When the purines get broken down by the body, uric acid is produced and, if you suffer from gout, crystals of this uric acid can form in the kidneys and joints.

Oddly enough, olive oil (the only oil in the Mediterranean diet) contains no omega-3s. Its main constituent is oleic acid, which belongs to the less beneficial omega-9s. It is a bit of a mystery, but research is ongoing into the undoubted benefits of olive oil. It certainly seems to have marked anti-inflammatory effects.

Avoid junk food

Junk food seems to promote inflammation. By 'junk food', I mean 'fast food' with added fat, sugar and salt, and processed foods with lots of additives.

The fact is that the trans fats and saturated fats used in preparing junk food and processed food certainly promote inflammation. Diets high in sugar have also been associated with increased inflammation, as well as predisposing you to obesity and diabetes. It is worth eliminating high-sugar foods such as fizzy drinks, pastries, pre-sweetened cereals and confectionery. It doesn't mean that you shouldn't have them as treats. Just don't have them regularly.

Omega oils are anti-inflammatory

The fact that the omega oils in the Mediterranean diet are anti-inflammatory associates them with a reduction in health risk, and recent research in the USA has shown that when people eat cholesterol-lowering foods in addition to going on a low-fat diet they can reduce their bad cholesterol by 13 per cent, as opposed to a mere 3 per cent when they only reduce the fat content. The beneficial foods are those containing plant sterols, such as nuts, foods with viscous fibre (including barley and oats), and soy protein, as in soya milk, tofu and soy meat substitutes.

Obesity

Go back to Chapter 10 if you want to recap on the health risks associated with obesity. If you need help with weight control, your doctor or practice nurse can advise you. Alternatively, there are several organisations like Weight Watchers and Slimming World, which can help in a group situation, wherein you try to lose weight along with other people.

A HEALTHY DIET AND TAKING SOME EXERCISE

Salt intake

I mention this here, since one's salt intake may have a direct bearing on blood pressure levels. As blood pressure is a risk factor for cardiovascular disease, it is therefore worth restricting your salt intake. The fact is that salt helps to push blood pressure up, by affecting internal regulatory mechanisms that push the pressure higher.

One of the main kidney functions is to remove unwanted fluid from the body. They do this by filtering the blood that flows through them and passing the unwanted fluid into the bladder. This is known as osmosis, the success of which depends on a delicate balance between the sodium and potassium levels in the blood. Osmosis causes water to be drawn out of the blood into collecting channels in the kidneys and these channels all drain into the ureters, the tubes that lead from the kidneys to the bladder.

If you take excess salt (sodium chloride) in your diet, you can alter the amount of sodium in your blood and this will in turn disrupt the kidneys' ability to maintain the mechanism of removing water from the blood. This will tend to cause the blood pressure to rise.

You must appreciate that blood pressure is very important. It is a real risk factor for strokes, heart failure and heart attacks. Sodium seems to be the culprit, and since salt is the main source of sodium in the diet it is the obvious thing to reduce to minimise your risk.

Adults are advised to consume no more than 6 g of salt a day. That is about a teaspoon. The average intake in the UK is about 9 g, 50 per cent more than is recommended. And for a large number of people who already have raised blood pressure, that is a very significant increase.

When you look at labels on food you must not assume that the sodium level that is given is the same as the salt level. To get the actual salt level, multiply the sodium level by 2.5.

Antioxidants

These are natural chemicals that are involved in the prevention of cell damage (the common pathway for inflammation), ageing and a whole host of degenerative diseases. They do this by mopping up free radicals, which are the culprits that cause the problems.

In many metabolic processes where oxidation takes place, free radicals are produced. These are atoms or groups of atoms with an odd number of unpaired electrons. These are very reactive radicals that can start chain reactions, in the way that rows of dominos tumble into one another. The end result is damage to cell components, such as the DNA and the cell membranes. You can think of this as being rather like leaving a rubber band exposed to the air for a long time; it becomes friable and frayed. If you think of that happening to cell membranes, the insides of vessels and the tissues of the back, then you can see how the effects can be far-reaching.

Everyone knows that you should eat five pieces of fruit or vegetable a day. It sounds simple, but a lot of people never manage that much. It is even better to eat your five a day 'the colour way', by eating five pieces of different-coloured fruit and vegetable. And if you do that you will be taking in a healthy supply of antioxidants, which will help reduce inflammation.

Five fruit and veg a day – eat the rainbow way

It is well established that eating five portions of fruit or vegetable every day can reduce your risk of heart disease and stroke, and also of certain cancers. The reason that they are so beneficial is because they are rich in antioxidants.

By varying the colours that you take you can get even more benefit, by getting the widest range of healthy nutrients. Use the rainbow as a loose guide:

Red fruit and vegetables are good sources of the nutrients lycopene, ellagic acid and quercetin. Tomatoes are rich in lycopene, which is known to be beneficial for men's prostate health and is also protective to the heart. Ellagic acid is abundant in raspberries, strawberries and pomegranates. It is a powerful antioxidant that seems to have anti-cancer properties, and is especially protective to the bowel. Apples are rich in quercetin, another antioxidant, which helps the body deal with allergens. Recently it has been found to help asthma.

Yellow and orange fruit and vegetables contain beta-carotene, flavonoids and lycopene. Beta-carotene is converted into vitamin A by the liver. It is good for eye health and has a beneficial effect on eyesight. In addition, it has been shown to decrease cholesterol levels in the liver. Think of adding apricots, oranges, lemons, peaches, papayas and pineapples to your weekly fruit shopping. And sweetcorn, peppers and butternut squashes.

Green fruit and vegetables have so much goodness it is hard to know where to start. The nutrients found in these vegetables reduce cancer risks, lower blood pressure and bad cholesterol levels, help the function of the digestive tract, support retinal health and vision, and boost the immune system.

Blue and purple fruit and vegetables, including prunes, grapes and raisins, are rich in flavonoids, which boost the immune system and are anti-inflammatory. Blueberries are particularly rich in lutein, which has been shown to be good for eye health, especially in the middle-aged and elderly. In addition, it is beneficial for the heart. Aubergines are rich in B vitamins, plus potassium, iron and zinc. It is another good one for prostate health. About a third of an aubergine would count as a portion.

White fruit and vegetables contain nutrients such as beta-glucans and lignans that boost the immune system. They activate B and T cells, the natural germ killers that are thought to reduce the risk of colon, breast and prostate cancers. There is some evidence that they also help to balance hormone levels, reducing the risk of hormone-related cancers. Here you can think of bananas, pears, white nectarines, garlic, onions, cauliflowers and mushrooms.

Potatoes are pretty much a mainstay of the British diet. But unfortunately they do not count towards the five a day. Nor do yams or cassavas, because they are all starchy food. So, it is good to try to get make vegetables a bigger part of a meal, and not just a little something to add to the plate beside the meat and the potatoes. That is why thinking of the colours of the rainbow (and white) might help.

Take some exercise

It is well established that even occasional exercise reduces the risk of cardiovascular disease. Regular exercise three or four times a week certainly reduces the risk further. The benefits of exercise are many, including:

- Strengthens your heart and circulation
- Helps heart failure
- Helps lower blood pressure
- Improves muscle strength and tone
- Strengthens bone
- Makes you fitter
- Lifts your mood.

If you have had a heart attack then you will have been advised about this as part of the cardiac rehabilitation programme that you went on. If you have not had a heart attack, but have not taken exercise for a while either, then see your doctor for a blood pressure recording and advice on how much exercise you can safely take to start. He or she can also advise you about incorporating the timing of your medication into your exercise schedule.

Types of exercise

There are three basic types:

Stretching

This is very important, since it is easy to pull or strain a muscle if you exercise without having 'warmed up'. This is especially the case with more energetic exercises, so stretching should always be built into your programme. Stretching arms and legs before activity helps to prepare the muscles (18 seconds is necessary to actually do a stretch, so 20 seconds makes sure you have stretched adequately). For any running activity, be sure to stretch the quads and the calf muscles:

- *Quadriceps* – stand and secure your balance by holding on to a table or window ledge or suitable thing. Then raise one leg backwards and bend the knee. Take hold of the foot and bring it up as close as you can to the bottom. Hold it there for 20 seconds and then relax. Do the other leg.

- *Calf muscles* – stand about a yard from a wall and keep one leg straight with both feet flat on the ground. Bend the other leg at the knee and lean forward against the wall. You will feel the straightened calf feel slightly taut. Hold this for 20 seconds then relax. Do the other side.

Cardiovascular or aerobic exercises

These include walking, jogging, skiing, rowing, tennis, golf, etc. Basically, it is any steady exercise in which you use large muscle groups. As the name implies, it exercises heart and lungs. If it is done over a period of time it will strengthen the heart and lower the blood pressure.

Strengthening exercises

These are exercises designed to build muscles, i.e. lifting exercises that are done repetitively until a muscle is tired. These are not a good idea if you have heart failure. And you must not do any strenuous excise in the first eight weeks after a heart attack. Again, be guided by your doctor or cardiac nurse as to how much you can safely do.

It is not necessary to work out in a gym; you can exercise in your own home. Aim at 20 to 30 minutes three or four times a week (unless otherwise advised by your doctor or nurse).

And don't forget about housework

Research in 2005 at Indiana University in the USA shows that adults with high blood pressure may be able to lower it by carrying out cumulative tasks like raking leaves, going for brisk walks and doing housework.[19] Cumulative activities like these were shown to have a profound activity on the circulation.

The team looked at eight adults with normal blood pressure, ten adults with prehypertension and ten adults with established hypertension. They defined hypertension as being as a blood pressure above 140/90, and prehypertension as being between 120/80 and 140/90. All participants were asked to add cumulative activities as above to their daily routine. For 12 hours afterwards, they had their blood pressures measured. Overall, the extra activities resulted in an average drop of 7 points in the prehypertension group and 13 points in the established hypertension group. This is fascinating, since it implies an immediate effect. But not only that, the lower levels persisted after that, only gradually returning to the pre-activity levels.

The overall message is clear. Adding physical activities to the day, like extra housework, going up stairs rather than taking lifts, or walking to the postbox, all help to keep you healthy.

Finally, it is not all doom and gloom

A heart attack is a frightening thing to happen, but if the heart-attack survivor can accept it for what it is, a warning, then he or she, together with their doctor, can do a lot to reduce the risk of having another one. Many people turn their lives around, give up injurious and damaging habits and refocus their lives.

Appendix

Cardiopulmonary resuscitation (CPR)

You can save someone's life if you can perform CPR. It is done if someone is not breathing and his or her heart has stopped. It is a first aid technique that involves chest compressions and rescue breaths. The aim is to keep the circulation of blood going and to keep oxygen flowing to the brain and heart.

The idea of giving mouth-to-mouth resuscitation may not appeal if there is no facemask, or if you have not learned how to do it. In that case, simply doing chest compressions until help arrives will do.

First, if you come across a collapsed person, ensure that it is safe for yourself to touch the person. This is particularly important if you suspect that they have received an electric shock. Don't put yourself at risk.

If the person is not breathing and has no pulse, call 999 or 112, asking for an ambulance for a collapsed person who has no pulse and is not breathing, and giving your location. Then start CPR.

To give a chest compression put the heel of one hand on the breastbone, then place the other hand on top and interlock your fingers.

Use your body weight (rather than just your arms) to compress the chest. Press down about five centimetres at a time and aim to give fairly rapid heart compressions, a rate of about 100–120 per minute. That is about two compressions per second.

Do 30 compressions, and then give two rescue breaths into the mouth. To do this, gently tilt the head back and raise the chin with two fingers. Pinch the nose, put your mouth over theirs and blow so that the chest rises.

If there is someone to help, then after a few cycles, swap over and continue 30 compressions, then two rescue breaths, until help arrives.

As soon as they start breathing or they have a pulse, stop the CPR.

It is worth taking a first aid course to learn how to do this life-saving technique using mannequins.

Glossary

acetylsalicylic acid – the chemical name for aspirin.

aldosterone – a hormone released by the adrenal gland which causes the kidneys to retain sodium and water.

angina – extremely tight chest pain caused when the heart is deprived of blood and therefore of oxygen.

angioplasty – a procedure in which a catheter is inserted into a groin (or wrist) artery and passed up into the heart in order to inflate a small balloon to open up the vessel. It may be combined with placing a stent, to keep the vessel open after the procedure.

angiotensin I – a protein involved in regulating blood pressure as part of the renin-angiotensin-aldosterone system.

angiotensin II – a powerful vasoconstrictor involved in regulating blood pressure as part of the renin-angiotensin-aldosterone system.

angiotensinogen – a peptide manufactured by the liver and involved in regulating blood pressure as part of the renin-angiotensin-aldosterone system.

anticoagulant – a drug to prevent blood coagulation. Warfarin, rivaroxaban and dabigatran are examples.

antiplatelet – a drug, such as aspirin, which prevents platelets from sticking together.

arrhythmia – an irregularity of the heartbeat.

arteriosclerosis – hardening of the arteries caused by accumulation of atheroma (same as atherosclerosis).

artery – blood vessel that carries oxygenated blood away from the heart, taking it to specific organs.

aspirin – the common name for acetylsalicylic acid, an antiplatelet agent that thins the blood and may be given to prevent a stroke.

asystole – the heart stops beating and electrical activity stops.

atheroma – fatty changes in a blood vessel.

atherosclerosis – hardening of the arteries caused by accumulation of atheroma.

atrial fibrillation – an irregular beating of the heart caused by loss of the heart's normal pacemaker, the sinoatrial node.

atrioventricular node – a special node in the middle of the heart which transmits electrical impulses down the two bundles of His to cause the ventricles to beat with each heartbeat.

bradyarrhythmia – an abnormal rhythm at a slow heart rate.

bradycardia – slow heart rate.

brain natriuretic peptide (BNP) – a protein that is raised in the blood in heart failure.

bundles of His – specialised conducting tissues that descend in the inter-ventricular walls (between the ventricles) to carry the wave of excitation from the atrioventricular node.

CABG – coronary artery by-pass graft operation done to improve the blood supply to the heart.

cardiac arrest – the heart stops beating. Unless it is quickly restarted, brain damage or death will swiftly follow.

cardiac effusion – an accumulation of fluid within the two layers of the pericardium.

cardiac tamponade – a life-threatening condition when a cardiac effusion is so extensive that it prevents the heart from beating.

cardiomyopathy – disease of the heart muscle. Cardiomyopathy is distinct from ischaemic heart disease.

cardiovascular disease – disease affecting the heart and the blood vessels, which can result in heart attacks, strokes and death.

catheter ablation – a procedure used to destroy an area of heart muscle that is causing an arrhythmia.

cerebrovascular disease – disease of the blood supply to the brain.

CHADS2 – an algorithm used for calculating the risk of having a stroke for patients with non-valvular atrial fibrillation.

cholesterol – a blood lipid or fat. There are two main types: LDL (bad) cholesterol and HDL (good) cholesterol.

clopidogrel – an antiplatelet agent that thins the blood and may be given to prevent a stroke.

coronary angiogram – a procedure in which a catheter is inserted into the heart via an artery and dye is injected. This gives a view of the coronary arteries to see if any blockages are present.

coronary thrombosis – blood clot forming in a coronary artery.

COX enzymes – cyclooxygenase enzymes, involved in producing prostaglandins and thromboxane. Aspirin blocks their effect.

cyanosis – blue or purple discolouration due to lack of oxygen.

DVT – a deep-vein thrombosis.

diabetes mellitus – a disorder of carbohydrate metabolism from too little insulin, or from an inadequate response to the body's own insulin.

dipyridamole – an antiplatelet agent that thins the blood and may be given to prevent a stroke.

echocardiogram (or ECHO) – a test using sound waves to build up a picture of the heart as it beats.

electrocardiogram (or ECG) – a test to measure the electrical activity of the heart.

endocardium – the lining of the heart and the heart valves.

heart failure – failure of the heart to maintain the circulation.

hepatomegaly – enlargement of the liver.

homoeostasis – the body's ability to control its internal workings and inner environment.

homocystinuria – a genetic condition in which raised levels of an amino acid carries an increased risk of coronary heart disease.

hypercholesterolaemia – raised blood cholesterol.

hyperkalaemia – raised potassium level.

hypokalaemia – low potassium level.

infarction – permanent damage to tissue after cells have died, leaving behind scar tissue.

inflammation – the process whereby the body tries to deal with injury and infection.

INR (international normalised ratio) – a blood test used to check on the dosage of warfarin needed.

ischaemia – deprivation of tissue of oxygen.

Korotkoff sounds – the sounds that can be heard with the stethoscope when listening over the brachial artery in the arm while measuring blood pressure.

left ventricular hypertrophy (LVH) – enlargement and thickening of the wall of the left ventricle.

lumen – the space in a blood vessel through which blood flows.

morphine – a major opiate drug, often used to relieve the pain of a heart attack.

myocardial infarction – a heart attack, resulting in damage to or death of part of the myocardium or heart muscle.

myocardial ischaemia – state in which the myocardium, the heart muscle, is deprived of blood and therefore of oxygen.

myocarditis – inflammation of the myocardium, the heart muscle.

myocardium – the heart muscle.

necrosis – the process of cell and tissue death.

NSTEMI – non-ST elevation myocardial infarction, whereby the arterial supply is only partially blocked off, so only part of the heart muscle is damaged.

papilloedema – swelling of the optic discs in the eyes, which can occur in severe malignant hypertension.

pericardium – the two-layered sac that envelops and anchors the heart.

pericarditis – inflammation of the pericardium.

plaque – fatty streaks inside an artery. They may rupture, causing an inflammatory reaction and the start of a clot.

platelet – the smallest type of blood cell. It does not contain DNA. Its function is to clump with other platelets to form a clot to plug a bleeding vessel and help heal a wound.

prostaglandin – natural hormones that are involved in many body processes, including pain, tissue injury and inflammation.

pulmonary circulation – the circulation to the lungs.

pulmonary embolism – when an embolism from a DVT lodges in a lung vessel.

Purkinje system – a network of specialised conducting tissues in the ventricle walls, which spreads a wave of excitation that causes the ventricles to contract.

renin – a hormone released from the kidney involved in regulating blood pressure as part of the renin-angiotensin-aldosterone system.

Ross procedure – this involves replacing the patient's aortic valve with their own pulmonary valve, then replacing the pulmonary with an artificial tissue valve.

Stokes-Adams attacks – these are faints due to insufficient blood being pumped to the brain.

STEMI – ST elevation myocardial infarction. This is a myocardial infarction with complete blockage of the blood supply to part of the heart muscle.

GLOSSARY

stenosis – a narrowing of an artery.

stent – a tiny wire tube that is placed inside a narrowed artery after an angioplasty in order to keep the vessel open.

systemic circulation – the circulation to the rest of the body apart from the lungs.

tachyarrhythmia – an abnormal heart rhythm at a fast heart rate.

tachycardia – fast heart rate.

thromboembolism – blood clot formation in a vessel which can potentially fragment to release a piece of clot (embolus). That broken clot could then lodge in a distant blood vessel as an embolism.

thrombosis – the process of blood clotting.

thromboxane – a chemical released by the action of COX-1 in platelets, causing them to clump and stick together.

thrombus – blood clot.

vein – blood vessel that returns blood to the heart.

white coat syndrome – the phenomenon that some people's blood pressure goes up when they see a health practitioner.

Directory of useful addresses

Blood Pressure UK

Blood Pressure UK, previously known as the Blood Pressure Association, is the UK charity dedicated to lowering the nation's blood pressure to prevent disability and death from stroke and heart disease. This charity offers a range of booklets, magazines, e-newsletters, a website, information line and other activities, to help people take control of, or prevent, high blood pressure.

Wolfson Institute
Charterhouse Square
London
EC1M 6BQ
Tel: 020 7882 6255 / 5793
Website: www.bloodpressureuk.org

British Cardiac Patients Association

The British Cardiac Patients Association (BCPA), previously known as The Zipper Club, is a non-profit-making organisation run by volunteers and established to provide support to cardiac patients and their carers. They offer advice and information about heart attack, angina, cardiac investigations, arrhythmias, stents, implantable cardiac devices, cardiac surgery for bypass, valve replacement, aneurysm, hole-in-the-heart, heart transplant or heart and lung transplant.

BCPA Head Office
15 Abbey Road
Bingham
Nottingham
NG13 8EE
Tel: 01949 837070
Website: www.bcpa.co.uk

British Heart Foundation

Funds raised by the BHF are used in the research and promotion of education about all issues arising from heart disease.

Greater London House
180 Hampstead Road
London
NW1 7AW
Tel: 020 7554 0000
Website: www.bhf.org.uk

The British Hypertension Society

A forum for professionals working in the field of hypertension and cardiovascular disease in the UK and Ireland. The society comprises doctors, nurses and other healthcare workers specialising in the delivery of care in hypertension and allied fields, together with clinicians and scientists in the forefront of cardiovascular research. The Society also provides a broad spectrum of scientific and educational activities, which include the production and regular updating of internationally renowned guidelines for the management of hypertension; an information service for healthcare professionals; and a validation service for manufacturers of blood pressure monitors.

c/o Hampton Medical Conferences Ltd
Rapier House
4–6 Crane Mead
Ware
Hertfordshire
SG12 9PW
Website: www.bhsoc.org
Email: bhs@le.ac.uk

The Cardiomyopathy Association

The Cardiomyopathy Association (CMA) is a registered charity that provides information and support to families affected by the heart muscle disease cardiomyopathy. It provides easy-to-understand information on the different types of cardiomyopathy. They have a freephone helpline (0800 0181 024) that is manned from 8.30 a.m. to 4.30 p.m. on weekdays.

Unit 10
Chiltern Court
Asheridge Road
Chesham
Bucks
HP5 2PX
Tel: 01494 791224
Helpline: 0800 018 1024 (freephone; Monday to Friday, 8.30 a.m. to 4.30 a.m.)
Fax: 01494 797199
Website: www.cardiomyopathy.org

Citizens Advice Bureau (CAB)

The Citizen's Advice Bureau aims to provide the advice people need for the problems they face, and to improve the policies and practices that affect people's lives. It provides free, independent and confidential advice. Advice by phone is available from all CAB offices and a national phone service is in development.

For Wales call 08444 77 20 20
For England call 08444 111 444
TextRelay users should call 08444 111 445

Disabled Living Foundation

DLF is a national charity that provides impartial advice, information and training on daily living equipment.

380–384 Harrow Road
London
W9 2HU
Helpline: 0845 130 9177 (textphone 020 7432 8009)
Email: helpline@dlf.org.uk

Drivers Medical Group
DVLA

Provides information about driving, licensing and medical conditions affecting driving.

Swansea
SA99 1TU
Tel: 0300 790 6806 (car or motorcycle) (Monday to Friday, 8 a.m. to 5.30 p.m; Saturday, 8 a.m. to 1 p.m.)

Tel: 0300 790 6807 (bus, coach or lorry) (Monday to Friday, 8 a.m. to 5.30 p.m; Saturday, 8 a.m. to 1 p.m.)
Fax: 0845 850 0095

HEART UK

HEART UK is an acronym. It stands for Hyperlipidaemia Education and Atherosclerosis Research Trust UK. It is a charity which will advise about cholesterol, lipid testing and interpretation of results. They can provide information, support and education, and they campaign for improved identification and standards of care.

Helpline: 0845 450 5988 (Cholesterol helpline open Monday to Friday, 10 a.m.–3 p.m. *Punjabi, Urdu & Hindi spoken on Friday.)*
Email: ask@heartuk.org.uk
Website: www.heartuk.org.uk

NHS Blood and Transplant

NHS Blood and Transplant (NHSBT) is a Special Health Authority, dedicated to saving and improving lives through the wide range of services we provide to the NHS. Our ambition is to be the best organisation of our type in the world.

Head Office
Oak House
Reeds Crescent
Watford
Hertfordshire
WD24 4QN
For NHSBT enquiries please contact:
Tel: 0300 123 23 23
Website: www.nhsbt.nhs.uk

NHS Smokefree

Advice about stopping smoking, including how to get help locally.

Tel: 0800 022 4332 (Monday to Friday, 9 a.m. to 8 p.m.; Saturday and Sunday 11 a.m. to 4 p.m.)
Website: www.smokefree.nhs.uk

NICE

The National Institute for Health and Care Excellence was set up in 1999 to reduce variation in the availability and quality of NHS treatment and care. NICE issues evidence-based guidance on the management of various conditions, and public health guidance recommending the best ways to encourage healthy living, promote wellbeing and prevent disease. It is funded by the Department of Health.

Website: www.nice.org.uk

Transplant Support Network

This is a telephone support network to help and support transplant patients and their families and carers throughout Britain.

Tel: 0800 027 4490/0800 027 4491
Email: admin@transplantsupportnetwork.org.uk

References

1 Doll, R. & Hill, A. B. Smoking and Carcinoma of the Lung: preliminary report. *BMJ* 221, 1950; 739–748.

2 Doll, R. & Hill, A. B. The Mortality of Doctors in Relation to Their Smoking Habits: a preliminary report. *BMJ* 228, 1954; 1451–1455.

3 Doll, R. & Hill, A. B. Lung Cancer and Other Causes of Death in Relation to Smoking: a second report on the mortality of British doctors. *BMJ* 233, 1956; 1071–1076.

4 Hurlbutt, F. R. Peri Kardies: A Treatise on the Heart from the Hippocratic Corpus, introduction and translation, *Bulletin of the History of Medicine*, 1939; (7), 1104–1113.

5 Katz, A. M. & Katz, P. Diseases of the Heart in the Works of Hippocrates, *British Heart Journal* 1962; 24:257–264.

6 Souter, K. Doctor's *Latin – A Miscellany of Latin and Greek Phrases* (2006, Robert Hale).

7 The Hypertension Trust

8 Acierno, L. J. *The History of Cardiology* (1994, The Parthenon Publishing Group); 493–500.

9 Acierno, L. J. *The History of Cardiology* (1994, The Parthenon Publishing Group); 110.

10 Ramrakha, P. & Hill, J. *Oxford Handbook of Cardiology* (2012, Oxford University Press); 368.

11 WHO figures as reported on NationMaster.com, a database source drawing on the CIA World Factbook and on UN, WHO and OECD facts and statistics www.nationmaster.com/graph/hea_hea_dis_dea-health-heart-disease-deaths.

12 Ramrakha, P. & Hill, J. *Oxford Handbook of Cardiology* (2012, Oxford University Press); 224.

13 Ashwell, M., Gunn, P., Gibson, N. Waist-to-height ratio is a better screening tool than waist circumference and BMI for adult cardiometabolic risk factors: a systematic review and meta-analysis. *Obesity Review*, 2012; 275–286.

14 Keatinge, W. R., Coleshaw, S. R., Cotter, F., Mattock, M., Murphy, M. & Chelliah, R. Increases in platelet and red cell counts, blood viscosity and arterial pressure during mild surface cooling: factors in mortality from coronary and cerebral thrombosis in winter. BMJ (Clinical Research Edition), 1984; 289 (6456):1405–1408.

15 Souter, K. *An Aspirin a Day – the Wonder Drug That Could Save Your Life* (2011, Michael O'Mara).

16 Peters, R. J., Mehta S, Yusuf, S. Acute coronary syndromes without ST segment elevation. *BMJ*, June 16, 2007; 334(7606): 1265–9.

17 Wexler, R. Ambulatory blood pressure monitoring in primary care. *Southern Medical Journal*, May 2010; 103(5): 447–52.

18 Sytkowski, P. A., Kannel, W. B., D'Agostino, R. B. Changes in risk factors and the decline in mortality from cardiovascular disease. The Framingham Heart Study, *New England Journal of Medicine*. June 7, 1990; 322(23): 1635–41.

19 Padilla, J., Wallace, J. P., Park, S. Accumulation of Physical Activity Reduces Blood Pressure in Pre- and Hypertension. *Medicine & Science in Sports & Exercise, Volume 37*, 2005;1264–1275

Have you enjoyed this book?
If so, why not write a review on your favourite website?

If you're interested in finding out more about our books,
find us on Facebook at **Summersdale Publishers** and
follow us on Twitter at **@Summersdale.**

Thanks very much for buying this Summersdale book.

www.summersdale.com